DESIGNED TO ADAPT

LEADING HEALTHCARE IN CHALLENGING TIMES

By John Kenagy, MD, MPA, ScD, FACS

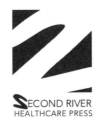

SECOND RIVER
HEALTHCARE PRESS

DESIGNED TO ADAPT:
Leading Healthcare in Challenging Times

By John W. Kenagy, MD, MPA, ScD, FACS

Second River Healthcare Press
26 Shawnee Way, Suite C
Bozeman, MT 59715
Phone (406) 586-8775 | FAX (406) 586-5672

Editor: Michelle Nash
Cover Layout & Design: Lan Weisberger
Typesetting/Composition: Neuhaus/Tyrrell Graphic Design

Kenagy, John   *Designed to Adapt: Leading Healthcare in Challenging Times/*
John Kenagy

Includes bibliographical references

ISBN-10: 0-9814605-2-6 *(hard cover)*   ISBN-10: 0-9814605-3-4 *(soft cover)*
ISBN-13: 978-0-9814605-2-9 *(hard cover)*   ISBN-13: 978-0-9814605-3-6 *(soft cover)*

1. Healthcare Management
2. Quality and Process Improvement
3. Leadership Development

Library of Congress Control Number: 2009924544

First Printing: September 2009

Second River Healthcare Press books are available at special quantity discounts. Please call for information at: (406) 586-8775 or order from the websites:

www.SecondRiverHealthcare.com
www.DesignedToAdapt.com

TABLE OF CONTENTS

DEDICATION

To my parents, Sylvia and Wyman Kenagy;
my wife, Jonell Day Kenagy;
and my children, Jennifer Aroha Hawkins,
Susanne, Emma and John;
whose love and support
made it safe for me to learn to adapt.

FOREWORD

The Innovator's View

There are two critical pathways for improving the quality and reducing the cost of healthcare. The first pathway is disruptive innovation — technological and business model innovations that lower costs while simultaneously creating access to ever more sophisticated levels of care. My recent book, *The Innovator's Prescription*, summarizes the roles that disruptive innovations can play in transforming healthcare.

Dr. John Kenagy leads the second pathway, one of vast and untapped potential. I met John more than a decade ago. He had taken leave of his career as a physician and executive in a highly respected healthcare system in the Pacific Northwest to obtain a Masters Degree at Harvard's Kennedy School of Government.

In 1997, John crossed the Charles River to enroll in my Harvard Business School course, *Managing Innovation*. Instantly, he began teaching me how my theories of innovation could relate to improving healthcare. Seeing how his facile mind caught the connections, I supported his appointment as a Visiting Scholar at Harvard Business School and introduced him to Steven Spear, at that time a Harvard Business School doctoral candidate. Steve was helping Toyota understand that their success rested on their unique approach to managing complex, collaborative work.

Steve discovered the underlying DNA of the Toyota Production System; the unspoken Rules-In-Use that govern everyday work. His recent book, *Chasing the Rabbit*, tells the tale and, in my opinion, he is doing the world's best thinking on process improvement.

When John began to understand Steve's work, he saw much more than a powerful manufacturing system. He saw a unique way to manage the complex, dynamic, unpredictable work of healthcare. John has developed Adaptive Design to be the enabling technology and operating system that brings this knowledge to healthcare.

This is a powerful combination and the rest is becoming history.

Hundreds of lives and millions of dollars have already been saved as John, Steve, and John's associates teach healthcare administrators, physicians and staff how to design and improve their processes and manage the knowledge that is inherent in their organization.

However, as profound as these insights and achievements are, they have only influenced a fraction of those who could, and should, benefit. Now his concept of Adaptive Design begins to break a tradeoff that pervades the work of every established, leading organization.

We can't afford what healthcare costs today, yet we need more. It is a hand-wringing tradeoff between having better quality healthcare, lower-cost care, and more conveniently accessible care. The result? — politicians, employers, and frustrated healthcare reformers worldwide exasperatedly throw up their hands at the intractability of the healthcare problem, their anguish mirroring the facial and body language of the Burghers of Calais that Rodin captured in his timeless sculpture.

But does having more of one thing require compromising the others? Of course not. There is a solution. The problem is that it is a disruptive one, and my work has shown it is almost impossible for an established organization to address the disruptive market successfully. That's the tradeoff — keep doing what you know how to do, you'll keep getting what you currently get and find it almost impossible to do something different. In healthcare, that creates a tradeoff — increasing quality increases costs.

Kenagy's concept of Adaptive Design begins to break that tradeoff. John has discovered that Adaptive Design gives the original, core business far greater flexibility in adapting to the demands of the market than I had ever thought achievable. I said, "It's almost impossible." That's true. But it's not impossible. Dr. John Kenagy and Adaptive Design are truly expanding the possible for healthcare.

Together, these two pathways of innovation (disruptive innovation and Adaptive Design) have the potential, in my opinion, of greatly improving the quality of healthcare while reducing its cost by 50 percent or more. I am not overstating this potential and I am grateful to John Kenagy and his associates for bringing to bear their wonderfully insightful minds on this topic of global impact.

Clayton Christensen
Professor
Harvard Business School

INTRODUCTION

The Frontline View

D
r. John Kenagy has drawn on his years of medical experience and management research to clearly articulate a comprehensive model for improving healthcare. It's called Adaptive Design.

Kenagy's Adaptive Design provides a framework and common language for designing, doing and improving the complex work of healthcare. Because it can be understood and practiced at all organizational levels, it also enables a cultural shift that can transform any clinic, hospital or healthcare system.

Adaptive Design continually moves patient care toward Ideal by embedding the Scientific Method and structured problem solving into everyone's daily work. Starting in one small place (the Learning Line), this methodology emphasizes providing "Ideal Patient Care," everyday by everyone. Leadership and management, in turn, become the "Help Chain" to develop and support this frontline focus on excellence.

To put it simply, Kenagy's Adaptive Design method is an operating system focused on identifying when care is not "Ideal" as a problem to be solved as quickly and simply as possible. The role of management transitions from meetings, gathering data and implementing solutions, to developing and empowering the frontline to systemically solve those problems as they happen. The result? Safety increases while quality, efficiency and flexibility are guaranteed at continually lower cost.

Adaptive Design develops people, builds trust and optimism and provides new opportunities for innovation while simultaneously making a difference for patients. This kind of focus and self-reinforcing cycle of improvement is at the heart of what has made Toyota and other select organizations success-ful decade after decade.

Based on my Mayo Health System experience, I have one word for Kenagy's Adaptive Design model: *Brilliant.*

Mark Lindsay, MD
Quality Officer
Mayo Health System

PROLOGUE

Why This Book? Why Now?

When I started writing this book, my goal was to show how our struggling healthcare system could benefit from combining the strategy of *disruptive innovation* with the *leadership and management capabilities* of adaptive, transformational companies — particularly Toyota. Now, suddenly, times have changed.

As I pen this Prologue, it is no secret that the world has suddenly become a much different place.

The message is clear: Surviving is no longer just a struggle for a few. Facing the facts, we see that the financial systems of many developed countries are severely damaged. The U.S. healthcare system is out-of-balance, if not hopelessly broken. This, however, is not just an American problem. Every healthcare system in the developed world faces severe challenges of rising costs and diminishing access. And answers are not in sight.

These *are* challenging times. The tattered fabric of business, insurance, finance, healthcare and government inherited from the 20th Century is unraveling in the 21st.

While the ultimate consequences are unknown, one thing is certain: The world in which medicine and surgery are practiced and healthcare institutions are managed is rapidly changing in complex and unpredictable ways.

But, challenging times also present great opportunities. History is clear that, in periods of rapid change, highly adaptive organizations have great competitive advantage. They do wonderful things. And they make a difference!

This book is about how you (and others like you) can link together to make that difference. Each chapter describes and translates the real-life healthcare experiences that show how success in changing times is dependent on accepting and practicing three principles recognized by successful adaptive innovators:

1. Your future success is not dependent on what you have done in the past or are doing now, but rather on how you *adapt* what you are doing to a constantly changing environment. This is the *challenge*.

2. The structures and systems of your current organization and the habits, behaviors and values of the people embedded within them *always* slow, stall and usually stop adaptive change. This is the *warning*.

3. Those few organizations strategically and operationally "Designed to Adapt" have competitive advantage in a rapidly changing world (Adaptive Design). This is the *opportunity*!

The evidence is clear on *what* to do. To achieve lasting results means more than holding your ground, implementing best practices or just changing *things*, like strategic plans, facilities, people, processes, product lines, technology or organizational charts. Sustainable competitive advantage means changing minds and developing people to continually adapt to new opportunities.

Those are the facts. Now the hard part: *How* to do it. The difficulty is *always how* to consistently execute adaptive change in the face of organizational barriers and the inertia of people (e.g., staff, physicians, management, regulators, government, even patients) who don't want change. But there is a tested solution. As you will discover in this book, Adaptive Design is the proven "how-to" method for making a difference in healthcare.

Adaptive Design combines disruptive innovation strategy with the leadership and management methods of those few great companies (e.g., Toyota, Intel, Southwest Airlines) who have adapted. For example, while formerly stronger companies struggle and fail, Toyota builds new capability even in the worst of times. What's Toyota's "disruptive" secret? Surprisingly, it is not "better process improvement" but rather their unique *knowledge management* methods that are "designed to adapt." They build into their organizational DNA the capability to change minds and develop people to adapt and respond to complex, dynamic, unpredictable opportunities.

This book shows how that same adaptive capacity can work in your organization! While the chapters offer instruction on how to lead in challenging times, they are not targeting just senior management. In Adaptive Design, *everyone is empowered* and *everyone is accountable* for taking the lead in adapting his or her own corner of the organization to any and all new realities.

For healthcare, leading in challenging times means revitalizing trust, optimism, high performance and innovation that makes a difference for patients. Get patients exactly what they need at continually lower cost. It's the way to fix healthcare. That's everyone's job. It's a tough uphill journey, but together we can do it.

So, let's start the climb.

John Kenagy, MD

CHAPTER 1

THE CLIMB

"You can observe a lot by just watching."

– YOGI BERRA

How could an American-trained vascular surgeon transition to studying innovation at Harvard Business School and end up writing a book on the management methods of a Japanese car company?

My answer is simple: "I fell into it — literally!"

Summer of 1992, University of Washington, Seattle: I had just finished teaching a course in Advanced Trauma Life Support. In an irony of all ironies, I was the one about to be traumatized.

My family and I had planned a weekend of camping at the beautiful Penrose Point State Park on Puget Sound, 30 miles outside Seattle. After a picnic lunch near the park's Mayo Cove, my four-year-old son John begged me to climb a tree with him. My excuse for such nonsense was to "catch a panoramic view of the water." As I scrambled up after John, already high in the tree, I faintly recall hearing my wife say, "I hope when he falls, he doesn't break something."

A moment later, I slipped. And indeed I did break *something*: my neck. I would spend the next three months in a halo brace and another three disabled and in therapy.

I observed and learned a lot by just watching, because I couldn't do much else. Like other medical personnel who have suddenly landed in a

1

patient's role, the event was life-altering. Even beyond the emotional and physical trauma, my deepened understanding of serious issues involving healthcare was both a lightning bolt and a gradual awakening — like time-lapse nature cinematography of a flower from seed to full bloom.

Immediate was my understanding that many professionals were working long and hard to meet my needs as a patient and to ensure a positive clinical outcome — which they did. But there is more to this story than dedicated people trying harder to meet patient needs. This book will compress the time-lapse story of all the discoveries that led to the full bloom of Adaptive Design, a way to develop your internal resources to successfully manage and do the work of healthcare in troubled times.

From my hospital bed I had a perspective in a way I could never have imagined as a physician on the floor. Over the duration of my recovery I witnessed many providers and managers laboring on my behalf against a system that was more of a cumbersome albatross than a support mechanism. All too often the staff seemingly had to "move heaven and earth" to accomplish what was needed.

Was this experience unique to that particular hospital? Both my personal "laboratory" ordeal and peer-reviewed research says *no*.

In 2003, the *California Management Review*[1] published research from Harvard Business School that documents 239 hours of observing nurses at "the point-of-care" in nine different hospitals. I will refer to this great paper frequently throughout this book. The study's intent was to gain a clearer understanding of the root causes of system failures, and the conclusion cited two: **errors** and **problems**.

The good news was that the nurses made relatively few medical errors. The startling (bad!) news was that they encountered an enormous number of problems that got in their way of delivering care — most were system-based. A large number of the failures resulted from nurses either not having what they needed or running into on-site interferences, i.e., *something was missing or in the way.*

The problems clearly originated less often with people and more often with the system. Such statistics validated what I had experienced as a patient ten years earlier. During that surreal experience of having my head affixed to a stabilizing halo with bolts screwed to my skull, my mind was clear. And

---

1 Tucker & Edmondson. *Why Hospitals Don't Learn from Failures: Organizational and Psychological Dynamics that Inhibit System Change.* See the Annotated Bibliography arranged by chapter for all reference information.

what I observed changed the idealistic and somewhat naïve notions of healthcare I had harbored, as a doctor, up to that point.

For example, so many good folks working hard to get me what I needed, so many obstructions and delays getting in their way. Couldn't that somehow be fixed?

My conclusion: They could be fixed if hospitals were "managed" better. My resolution: Join management. Eventually, I filled the position of Regional Vice President for Business Development with a well-respected, multi-state, integrated health system in the Pacific Northwest, while maintaining my surgeon status.

Two things became clear during my five-year tenure juggling both clinical and administrative responsibilities:

1. Some of my hard-won, top-down contributions as an executive actually got in the way of my efforts as a physician trying to meet patients' needs — especially when we either redesigned the work with projects and technology or struggled to comply with regulations or tried to control costs.

2. What I required as a physician (basically more resources and flexibility) became a nightmare to me as a budget-strapped executive struggling to keep afloat in a turbulent sea of unexpected demands, unfunded mandates and diminishing resources.

I found myself trapped in the proverbial circular debate between two irreconcilable differences — or, caught "between a rock and a hard place." And neither option felt comfortable.

From the outside, our so-called "model" health system looked well positioned for the future. With all the attributes of an advanced managed care organization, e.g., an electronic medical record (EMR), employed, "integrated" physicians, our own health plan, the latest in process improvements, new state-of-the-art facilities and technology — basically we lacked nothing.

Internally, however, we struggled with increasing complexity, rising costs, declining reimbursement, decreasing staff and physician morale, and increasingly frustrated patients. As I searched the country for answers, to my chagrin I discovered that others were seemingly trying to get where we were. They didn't know that "where we were" was becoming increasingly difficult and challenging. And we weren't telling!

Blaming ourselves for the problems, we adopted the adage, "When the going gets tough, the tough get going." As such, the mantra for our executive team was simple: "Try harder." *But how?*

Desperately needing an understanding of why management, staff and physicians' best-intended efforts were failing, I sought an outside view — outside the West Coast and ultimately outside of healthcare.

I went to Boston, first to Harvard's Kennedy School, then across the Charles River to the Harvard Business School. There, I took on another title: Visiting Scholar. During that tenure, two innovative concepts generated a solution — eventually called Adaptive Design — that would forever change my vision and approach to healthcare.

Discovery number one came from the topsy-turvy world of "disruptive innovation." Professor Clayton Christensen, my sponsor at Harvard Business School, produced research showing that, when the world fundamentally changes, top companies of the day *almost never* lead in the transformation!

Entrapped by their own success, leading organizations and their management teams miss opportunities to create new products and services based on less complex ideas, fewer costly processes, and simplified technologies that don't match current methods and expectations. Christensen coined the term *disruptive innovation* to describe this unique phenomenon.

The history of disruptive innovation is the story of successful organizations missing the boat:

- "Bigger sailing ships are the future — not smoky, noisy, dangerous steam engines."
- "Why worry about telephones when our telegrams work so well!"
- "People want big cars with fins — not cheap, tiny imports."
- "Why bother with low cost shopping and malls? Our downtown department store is doing fine!"
- "Computers are for business. There is no place for a computer in the home."
- "Why change the way we manage our hospital? We have provided great care for years."
- "Why should I change how I care for patients? I'm a good doctor."

For me, the discovery of disruptive innovation was liberating. I could stop feeling guilty.

Ever since breaking my neck, I had been committed to improving care for patients. But despite years of "trying harder," I was still struggling to make a difference. The biggest hurdle was that I worked for a successful, leading healthcare organization. According to Christensen's great, counterintuitive insight, *I was unlikely to find the answers there.*

Since, during a transformation, the current leaders rarely lead the change, disruptive innovation gave me permission to look elsewhere. It even guided my first steps: Look for effective, simpler, less costly ways to provide better care — in places normally off the radar screen of established health-care leaders.

Still something was missing. Knowing *what* to do doesn't help, if you don't know *how* to do it.

That led to discovery number two: the *how* factor. But learning how to create and carry out a disruptive innovation did not come from some "magic kingdom" medical center, but from where I least expected: a Japanese car manufacturing company.

Toyota has been recognized for years as a great automobile company. Its manufacturing practices and improvement tools (described as *Lean Manufacturing*) are researched and generally well known. Hundreds of papers and books have been written (more than on any other company), and thousands of consultants and industry experts have implemented Toyota's best practices at great expense.

Completely transparent, Toyota shares what it does and how. The term "Lean" defines its powerful process-improvement tools. Many companies (including some in healthcare) have copied these Lean skills and tools to great success. But the mystery was that **no manufacturing company, unless directly taught by Toyota, ever duplicated its success.**

Professors Kent Bowen and Steven Spear at Harvard Business School set about to solve that mystery and learned that there was much more to the story than a great set of process-improvement tools. They taught me that four fundamental rules underlie the work of everyone at Toyota. Applying the rules to healthcare helped me understand that Toyota has a unique management system and business model that focuses on managing knowledge to develop every person in the organization. The focus is always on how to develop people to better meet customer needs.

Since more employees typically work at the frontline than in top management, most of the solutions to problems at Toyota come from the "bottom." In other words, the answers don't typically come from management, consultants or technology. And such incredible results don't happen by magic. Instead, Toyota's unique, adaptive knowledge management system makes it happen.

The discovery of Toyota's powerful people-developing, adaptive knowledge management system is exhilarating, because in my experience, healthcare's greatest strength is its people.

Most well-educated people have many employment opportunities, i.e., many ways to make money, gain power and control, and maintain a good job. But most of those in healthcare choose that career for another singular reason: the desire to care for others. They want to make a difference!

Imagine having management's main focus be to nurture, grow and develop people! For me that was a dream come true.

And then I woke up. I needed more than a new disruptive innovation strategy and a unique, adaptive knowledge management system. The combination of the two *had* to work together in healthcare.

That is the story of Adaptive Design — and the rest of this book.

Years of testing and improvement through the work of literally hundreds of dedicated people has led to Adaptive Design — the vision of transformational innovation tied to practical, new management methods that develop people as part of healthcare's daily work environment.

Adaptive Design is not disruptive innovation or the Toyota Production System; it's the combination and much more because it has been tested, validated and improved in the refining fire of the frontlines of healthcare. It is not in competition with Lean or other methods of process improvement because it is an adjunct and direct extension of their great and valuable work into a new place.

In this framework, there does not have to be a tradeoff between quality and cost in healthcare. Adaptive Design is an enabling technology that continually improves an organization's ability to deliver exactly what a patient needs while simultaneously lowering the cost of care.

This book proposes that the simple — but revolutionary — concept of Adaptive Design will change healthcare at its deepest level — forever.

Not only am I a surgeon, I am also a speaker, advisor, teacher and coach. In each role I offer a portrait of a revitalized, restructured, rejuvenated, patient-friendly healthcare system.[2] Such a vision has worked and will work, when all of us (policymakers, employers, educators, management, staff, physicians and patients) join hands and take the time to look, listen and learn; then test, validate and improve.

This work is not intended to be a textbook on Adaptive Design. Like

---

2 While this book targets healthcare, these concepts can be adapted to fit many other professions. Not long ago a schoolteacher told me, "I'm going to use disruptive innovation and Adaptive Design in my classroom." I suggested she write a book about the experience — and send me a copy!

other important skills, Adaptive Design can only be learned by doing. What this book will do is provide a framework for understanding the philosophy, principles, skills, tools, and methods fundamental to Adaptive Design.

In addition, I hope to provide an inspiring and refreshing reminder of healthcare's most valuable resource: people. After all, our business is caring. And caring is our business. Adaptive Design enables people to create (and recreate) business and care model innovations customized for our unique industry and our "most important customer:" the patient.

Granted, this isn't exactly the panoramic view I had in mind when I climbed that tree many years ago. But, my vision was changed forever. For that reason, I'll never regret the climb!

CHAPTER 2

WHY TOYOTA?

*"One of the greatest pains to human nature
is the pain of a new idea."*

– WALTER BAGEHOT

I literally had to break my neck to garner the initial research for this book. However, the issues raised here are so complex, so profound, and so *worthy* that I don't regret the pain nor lament the time lost. That said, I would not look forward to ever repeating such arduous "learning-by-doing."

Fortunately, you do not have to experience some traumatic odyssey to conclude that healthcare organizations must seek new opportunities to innovate and improve — *now*.

And a road map is available for getting there. It's called Adaptive Design.

The purpose of this book is to chart a path towards making a difference in healthcare by getting patients exactly what they need at continually lower cost. It's the way to fix healthcare.

Knowing we *can* is the important first step. In the context of Adaptive Design, leaders will experience the vision's reality in such improvements as:

- higher quality care,
- more flexibility and responsiveness to patient needs, and
- lower costs.

These are the guideposts: better care, patient focus and responsiveness, decreased costs. No tradeoffs! It's as simple as that.

Simple is not necessarily easy, however. That's a big order, so let's cut to the chase and answer a question that is probably on your mind: Why *Toyota*? Medical personnel care for people; Toyota makes cars. I often say, "Healthcare needs to lead like Toyota." So, what does that mean?

These contradictions were first posed to me many years ago during a seminar. In the midst of the "Managed Care Revolution" of the 1990s, I was presenting my early work with Toyota Production System methods to a sophisticated healthcare management team in California.

A physician shot-up during the Q & A segment and said, pointedly, "Hey, Kenagy, you're wrong. Dead wrong." (That's the thing about us physicians: We are so hesitant to speak our minds!) He continued on. "Your Toyota theories don't fit, because we do not practice medicine on assembly lines." Then he did a great imitation of a stiff-armed, mechanistic robotic worker picking up a box, rotating rigidly to his left, and setting down the box. In fact, he did it three times!

Then he finished with, "I am not a robot or an assembly line worker that you can pre-program to do some simple task. I am a *doctor*. I take care of *people*." With that he sat down, mission accomplished!

His words knocked me off my stride. After all, he was right. Healthcare employees are not industrial assembly line workers. So, is this analogy appropriate? My first answer for *"why Toyota"* is based on that company's unique, philosophically different approach to assembly lines.

Here's the story: For over 60 years Toyota factories have turned automobile manufacturing on its head. But their efficient productivity did not happen overnight. Nor did it happen without resistance from workers and managers wed to long-established practices. And it did not happen without revolutionary insights and learning.

In his book,[3] Taiichi Ohno describes how many of the production and business management techniques initially driving the Japanese auto industry came out of the U.S. auto empire. During the boom years of the 1960s, the Japanese auto industry prospered by copying American methods.

But Ohno, often identified as one of the originators of the Toyota Production System, writes: "We [at Toyota] kept reminding ourselves... that careless imitation of the American system could be dangerous."

America's manufacturing system was based on large-scale mass produc-

---

3 Taiichi Ohno. *Toyota Production System: Beyond Large-Scale Production.*

tion, i.e., maximize profit by producing a smaller selection of profitable products in large quantities. This is the classic "economies of scale," an industrial management model that almost all successful companies have followed over the last 150 years because it works. Such a model is unstoppable in times of prosperity. But Toyota's concern was valid: What would happen in hard times, such as recessions and economic downturns?

In the '60s and '70s, Toyota strategically changed its focus to a more flexible manufacturing system, sensitive to market forces. Out of that arose a unique production concept to *maximize profit by making limited numbers of a wide variety of products*. In doing so, Toyota turned the traditional model of economies of scale on its head.

The value of this paradigm shift was proven when hard times arrived — as they inevitably do. Toyota weathered the storm of the worldwide recession (triggered by the 1973 Oil Crisis) better and more profitably than more traditionally managed competitors, and they have never looked back.[4]

As such, Toyota developed an innovative, fundamentally new business model for manufacturing: Maximize profit by making limited numbers of many products. This focus is radically different than other traditional, industrial manufacturing enterprises.

Based on my experiences, that focus is also a great fit for healthcare.

Think of the number of products and services encountered in one evening at a typical busy community hospital emergency room. In my multiple observations of such settings, I can assure you that they run into the hundreds. Moreover, the scenario is completely unpredictable from night to night!

If you work in an ER, you know the typical scenario. You've just barely breathed the words "Boy, it's dead around here tonight..." when *whew*! — in scream the ambulances from the crash of a busload of hemophiliacs.

But, others say, "That's not representative. ERs are crazy places. Normal healthcare clinics or hospitals are more simple than that."

What about what a physician delivers from his or her office in one afternoon, which I have also observed. For example, let's spend two hours observing an internist in one of America's greatest health systems. In 120 minutes he sees eight different patients. That's not so bad, you say? Take a closer look:

Each patient has an average of four separate problems or complaints, usually entirely different from the admitting diagnosis. For example, one

---

4 As I finish this book, the downturn story is repeating itself with even greater intensity, and although Toyota is facing its first operating loss in more than 50 years, it is doing so from a vastly stronger position than its U.S. competitors.

patient's "headaches" turns out to be a potential anorexic and another's "feeling tired all the time" is actually a concern about a sexually transmitted disease.

In addition, the doctor actually only has 69 minutes of his two hours to spend with those patients. The other 51 minutes are spent documenting on a computer, hunting, fetching, interpreting, and clarifying what he needs for patient care and struggling with two different computers systems. (And all that in one of "America's Most-Wired" health systems.)

All these unpredictable circumstances are an everyday part of life in healthcare. In this book I will examine more deeply this complexity and how to manage it. Suffice it to say, healthcare delivers a huge number of unpredictable services daily — and, may I add, a job no robot (or computer) could ever do!

My conclusion: An industrial model patterned on economies of scale is a poor match for American medicine. On the other hand, an approach which allows an organization to flexibly and profitably produce small numbers of a wide variety of products and services is a better fit. That's the Toyota — and Adaptive Design — approach.

That's one reason "why Toyota!"

Let me add another reason that gets right back to the skeptical physician who mimicked a mechanical robotic — the part that involves people.

Toyota has, throughout its entire history, deeply embedded basic principles into its culture, its business model, and its people. These principles are extremely important to the company, so much that:

> [U]nder the presidency of Fujio Cho, Toyota embarked on an initiative to put into writing the wisdom of the founders that had been passed down verbally through all the generations. All of their sayings and anecdotes were collected and evaluated to form a set of values, beliefs, principles, insights, and intuitions for the company. In the process, two core values were identified as the pillars of *The Toyota Way 2001*: 'continuous improvement' and 'respect for people' based on the belief in [the power] of people's ordinary capabilities.[5]

Our traditional industrial management model makes much of Toyota's continuous improvement (kaizan), while mentioning Toyota's "respect for

---

5 Takeuchi H., Osono E., & Shimizu N. *Extreme Toyota.*

people" only in passing. In fact, this extraordinary respect for the ordinary capabilities of the average Toyota employee is, by their own description, one of the company's two great pillars.

Toyota's management states that "our number one resource is our people." And they prove it by, with great intentionality, respecting and developing each employee into an informed and capable "knowledge worker."[6]

A knowledge worker is the antithesis of the physician-skeptic's robot following programmed instructions and conforming to the rigid dictates of pre-designed work. Toyota knows that every employee has important, deeply held, experiential or tacit knowledge about what they do and how they do it. But this deeply held knowledge is not easily transferable to others.

Here's an example of what I mean. For readers who are managers, think of the many times you have met with your immediate supervisor, and then walked out of the meeting shaking your head and thinking, "He (or she) doesn't have the faintest idea of what I really do."

Every worker has tacit knowledge; the more complex the job, the harder it is to transfer this knowledge. For Toyota, the next step is for this ingrained, tacit knowledge to be developed further by converting it into explicit, transferable knowledge that benefits other workers, management and ultimately the customer.

To simplify, it's a two-tiered plan: (1) develop each worker's mind, work and skills in such a way that customers benefit, so, as a result, (2) the organization as a whole improves and thrives.

Try "programming" that into a robot!

"Respect for people" at Toyota translates into a company that has passed beyond the traditional industrial model dominating management for the past 150 years. Using healthcare as an example, notice the following philosophical extremes.

Under the industrial model, healthcare focuses on:

- managing processes,
- to coordinate and control people,
- to meet *management's* targets and goals.

---

6 "Knowledge worker" has been part of the argot of management terminology since the beginning of the "Information Age." Coined by the management guru Peter Drucker, for our purposes, a knowledge worker is a person who holds unique, tacit and difficult to transfer information about value-adding work that is imbedded into the context of what they are doing now. Knowledge management develops that individual's tacit knowledge and makes it available to others and the organization as a whole. For an original, perfectly applicable, but very non-healthcare view of the subject, see Friedrich Von Hayek's classic article on "The Use of Knowledge in Society," listed in the Bibliography. In addition, an Adaptive Design Glossary is included at the back of this book.

Clearly the focus is on process, control and products that meet goals.

As you will discover in this book, adapting the Toyota knowledge management model, Adaptive Design uses knowledge, training and the work itself:

- to develop people,
- to problem-solve systems,
- to achieve a unifying, common strategic purpose focused on the patient.

The focus is on people, problem solving and purpose.

So, back to "why Toyota?"

First, Toyota, in contradistinction to most industrially managed companies, seeks to make small numbers of a large variety of products and services. This is the opposite of traditional, deeply imbedded, mass-production focused, industrial management. Toyota's philosophy fits beautifully into the unique diversity and complexity of 21st Century healthcare.

Second, Toyota manufacturing has moved beyond the traditions and methods of industrial management. Their focus is not "process improvement." Their deep respect for people has led to the development of a unique, adaptive knowledge management system that is also a great fit for workers and management in healthcare.

As I teach healthcare organizations, I see these concepts transform the system time and time again.

The physician who buttonholed me with his question was exactly right. Healthcare workers are not robots. And it does not work to manage them as if they were!

So, that's the 10,000-foot panoramic view of "why Toyota?" The rest of the chapters will get down to earth with Adaptive Design in real-life healthcare. To hit the ground running, the next chapter shows what a hospital might look like two years after committing to adaptive management. It could be a hospital near you.

CHAPTER 3

THROUGH THE EYES
OF THE PATIENT

*"The pessimist complains about the wind; the optimist
expects it to change; the realist adjusts the sails."*

– WILLIAM ARTHUR WARD

Most everyone I know is pretty pessimistic about healthcare. Quite a few justifiably complain (sometimes loudly) that "Healthcare must transform — try harder!"

Even though I've usually been an optimistic person, after 38 years of trying harder, I am inclined to believe that the experts, pundits, and regulators who suggest that "trying harder" is the answer to healthcare transformation are unduly optimistic.

As in the quote above, I now lean towards the realist's approach and say it is time to trim the sails. It is time to *adapt.*

The great economist John Kenneth Galbraith, in his reflections on the future, said it well: "There are two kinds of people who tell us what is going to happen in the future: those who don't know and those who know they don't know." I think he may have something there. Perhaps trying to predict, design and implement the future may be part of our problem.

It seems to me that, under these circumstances, the adaptive realist has the advantage of being most able to respond to what's in the forecast. And history suggests it won't be a slow glacial process.

As a surgeon, healthcare executive, scholar and patient, I'll hedge my bets that some of us are already carving out a new future in healthcare. Answering the following single question could alone assure that possibility and accelerate the potential: *What would happen if a hospital started to get patients exactly what they needed at continually lower cost? Would that fix healthcare?* As an answer, allow me to present two scenarios...

Scenario A: Let's join a patient Bill, and his wife Ann, for a day at the outpatient surgery unit of St. Typical American Hospital ("St. TAH"), perhaps in a city near you, two years after St. TAH started down the Adaptive Design path toward Ideal Patient Care.

Bill Jones was not looking forward to his surgery at St. TAH. His chronic medical problem required recurrent outpatient surgeries, so he had "been there, done that" three times in as many years.

It's not that the surgery was so bad. Bill trusted the surgeon, and the discomfort was manageable. But after the last operation he had been laid-low by nausea. He also dreaded the hassles and frustration that had been part of his past healthcare experiences. In addition, because of recent local and national news reports documenting medical errors and stories of unnecessary hospital deaths, Bill was, quite frankly, concerned about his welfare.

Recalling last year's surgery didn't help. First, the operation had been delayed an hour. Then, although the procedure only took 30 minutes, Bill was very groggy and nauseated after the surgery and his recovery was slow, lengthening his stay to nearly six hours. His wife, Ann, had accompanied him, and they both found the day exhausting and stressful: long waits, obscure instructions and a harried medical staff who seemed to want to help but were always busy and distracted. This time Bill expected more of the same.

Despite his concerns, Bill had heard about changes at St. TAH. Word gets around, you know. Several friends had either been in the hospital or visited there recently — and they all swore that things had improved. But Bill and Ann were skeptical.

First off, they had a long-planned family reunion coming up, out of state. Bill needed the surgery before the trip, but he had forgotten to schedule it. Knowing that St. TAH was extremely busy, Bill dreaded having to plead with the scheduling coordinator to be worked in early. With trepidation, he dialed the number and hit the extension. Immediately he was referred to a nurse, Jane Smith.

"No problem," she said, in a friendly voice. Bill breathed a sigh of relief. Then Jane asked if next Friday at 2 P.M. would work. "That's almost too fast!" he thought, taken aback. And dare he suggest scheduling the surgery earlier in the day? "Don't worry," Jane responded. "We've learned a lot since your last visit. You should be ready for discharge by 4 P.M."

Bill couldn't believe his ears.

"I just need to confirm the information on your Ideal Health Card," continued Nurse Smith. "I see that you like your updated information sent by e-mail, so we'll do that."

The phone interview continued a few more minutes. At the end, Bill couldn't help but think, "That was refreshing." Was there ever a time he had a healthcare service scheduled so quickly or easily? Jane had even inquired about his wife by name, encouraging her to come to the procedure, along with other friends or family. Her questions and comments had certainly added to Bill's comfort level.

And that Ideal Health Card. During his last doctor's visit, Bill had his picture taken with a camera on a personal computer and was told the business office had simplified their data system. And after his appointment, he was handed a new, updated Ideal Health Card, with easy-to-follow instructions.

Bill could use the card to check in at any St. TAH's facility or associated physician's office and found it accomplished in seconds the irksome process of filling out another form on a clipboard or repeating the same information to a receptionist who stared more at the computer screen than at him.

The card worked for more than registration. Bill learned that it connected directly to the new medical savings account (MSA) that St. TAH had created in collaboration with his and several other local employers. Operating like a debit card, Bill used his Ideal Health Card to keep track of his deductible and co-pays, access specific information regarding *his* MSA, and connect with a new St. TAH's healthcare support group of other people with *his* medical condition.

Two days previous to Bill's surgery, Jane called to confirm his appointment and make sure he had received his pre-op instructions. Sure enough, they had arrived and were easy to understand. They even included a map with directions from Bill's house to the hospital, with approximate travel time. Based on these contacts, Bill was actually anticipating a positive hospital experience — for the *first time*.

But the day of his surgery did not look promising. It was pouring rain. Bill and Ann dreaded the drenching walk from the parking lot to the hospital or the wait for valet service. The map's instructions said, "Follow the yellow signs and park in A6." As soon as they got to the hospital grounds, yellow signs directed Bill to the specified parking lot for outpatient surgery. And *there*, a large A6 sign bearing his name identified his parking space—under cover and right next to the door!

The hospital was the same, but this convenient covered parking was all new.

When Bill and Ann walked through the door (dry!), they were immediately struck by improvements in design and décor. Bill had remembered the large, expansive lobby, lots of people, hustle and bustle, chairs filled with patients and family members — all *waiting*. (He and Ann had always joked sarcastically about the one constant in every medical experience — "the waiting room.")

Clearly, the lobby had been redesigned — smaller and simpler, bright and airy. Only two other people were visible, and one walked up to Bill immediately and said, "Hello, Mr. Jones. I recognize you from your Ideal Health Card. And this must be Mrs. Jones. Thanks for being right on time. My name is Jane Smith. I'll be your nurse today."

This was the same Jane Smith that Bill had been in contact with before. She took Bill and Ann back to a private consultation room, simple but tastefully decorated, and asked for Bill's Ideal Health Card. Passing it through a card reader, she reconciled the information (including medications) with Bill directly. Immediately, Bill realized he had not included a new medication recently prescribed by his doctor. Jane added the information into the computer and told Bill he would get a new card before leaving the hospital. "Good. You are all registered. Do you or Mrs. Jones have any questions about your surgery today?"

Bill and Ann were bubbling with questions, but not about the surgery. They wanted to know about the changes at St. TAH. "How can they provide all this personalized service?" Bill asked. Then, as he remembered stories of expensive healthcare "concierge" services, he added hesitantly: "We can't afford to pay anything extra."

Jane responded quickly. "The hospital didn't make these changes. We did. Management set the direction, taught us what to do, and challenged us to make it better. Pretty amazing, isn't it? Now, in 17 minutes I will take you back for your surgery. Unless you have more questions, I'll gladly tell you the story. Oh, and the cost will be less than last year. Working with your MSA and your company's health plan, we have reduced your co-pay and eliminated your deductible."

Amazed, Bill and Ann sat back to listen, all ears.

Jane described how two years ago St. TAH senior management had decided to try something different. They had heard about Adaptive Design — a way to streamline operations at a cost savings to both the hospital and the patient. After careful study, they went with the plan. The first step was to identify a place in the hospital to create a visionary environment that fostered trust, optimism, high performance and innovation. Hospital leadership chose outpatient surgery and called it St. TAH'S Learning Line.[7]

"None of us on the staff thought this would amount to anything new," Jane said. "In fact, I was deeply skeptical. And many were afraid this was just another way for management to lay off more people. But we quickly discovered how wrong we were."

Jane went on to describe how St. TAH brought in a team who wanted to learn from the staff and management how the place really worked. "What a difference from past consultants with their all-talk and no-listening.

"Through timely observations, they showed us diagrams and pictures of our typical work routines. We could see all sorts of waste, rework and redundancy in what we were doing. Add to that all the ambiguity, assumptions, workarounds and tradeoffs that got in our way — everywhere, everyday."

Bill responded, "Well, we certainly see a difference. Those consultants gave you some great solutions and wonderful new technology. Where did they get that Ideal Health Card idea? And my own parking space? And my own personal nurse?"

"Oh, that's the interesting part. The ideas didn't come from consultants. They came from us! Instead of putting together another task force and having a bunch of meetings, they taught us to signal when the system didn't provide what we needed to meet patient care needs Ideally. A manager was assigned the job of being our "designated problem solver" (they called her a Learner/Leader/Teacher), and we were encouraged to experiment with what might work best to eliminate those problems.

"Management told us we had one purpose to our work, 'Get patients exactly what they need at continually lower cost.' That's how we were going

---

7 Learning Line and Adaptive Design will be explained in detail later in the book. I will also refer back to Bill, Ann, and Jane. Meanwhile, think *"possibility"* as you continue with this story.

to do our part to fix healthcare.

"Therefore, from the start, management set direction by making it clear that we would be moving toward Ideal Patient Care — **exact, customized, immediate, safe** and **waste free**. All of us understood that right from the beginning, the patient was going to come first. We didn't know exactly how we were going to do it, but we had a purpose, a common direction, we would be moving forward and each of us understood where we were going!

"Another unexpected discovery was that we all had to follow certain rules if we wanted to improve. At first, based on our past experiences, everyone was afraid of more rules. But soon we discovered that the rules made it easier and safer to learn and improve. In the beginning, our work was pretty chaotic and inconsistent. We were definitely not delivering *Ideal* care. But we all had gone into healthcare to make a difference — and we *wanted* to improve patient care. When we found out that the rules made that easier, we all got on board."

It still didn't make sense to Bill. "But how about all these big changes? And you said you started two years ago. I was here a year ago. And not only did I not have any of these advantages, I had a pretty unpleasant experience."

Jane smiled and said, "We were starting to make some of the improvements you have experienced today. It was a matter of individuals partnering with simple technology to better meet your needs. At the start, it wasn't pretty. Your case last year was one of our big learning experiences."

"My case?"

"Your experience helped us begin to understand how solving our immediate problems and correcting our daily mistakes was a much more powerful way to improve than trying to implement somebody else's best practices or buy technology to design the 'perfect' system. Remember how sick you were after your surgery? That was a big learning point for us.

"The post anesthesia care unit (PACU) nurse signaled the problem. I remember the conversation: 'This just isn't right. He should have recovered and been on his way home long ago. But he's still nauseated, so I can't discharge him. The PACU is full, other patients are backed up in the OR, and now the whole surgery schedule is behind. This problem needs to be solved!'"

Bill responded, "But that's been going on for years. I've always been sick and slow to recover after surgery. What's going to be different this time?"

"In your case, the nurse signaled the problem to her designated support — her Learner/Leader/Teacher — and the anesthesiologists got involved immediately. Within days, a series of experiments began. You would be amazed what we learned from your case. Now our anesthesia management has been redesigned, and the communication between anesthesiologists, surgeons, nurses and management has dramatically improved.

"With these and hundreds of other small changes, we now use the same resources to care for many more patients. That's how management was actually able to lower charges. Higher quality and lower cost — that's not the way we used to work. Nobody wants to go back. Those were *not* 'the good old days.'

"In all truth, we nurses used to blame the doctors, while the doctors blamed us. We all blamed management, and management thought it was our fault. And everybody thought the real problem might be the patients — they were so demanding! Now, problems we struggled with for years are solved, often in a matter of hours, and rarely in more than a few days.

"Adaptive Design has shown us how obstacles are always system-problems, not people-problems. Today our care is not only more efficient and patient-centered, it is also much, *much* safer. Our problem solving has created a sustainable, blame-free culture of safety. Not only is no one blamed for identifying a problem, it is now clear that identifying problems and participating in problem solving is everyone's responsibility. And we take that responsibility very seriously. But, honestly, now we don't have to think about it much anymore. We just do it; it's part of our everyday work.

"Let me give you an example of how small things can make a difference," Jane continued. "Before Adaptive Design, our days were filled with workarounds. We got the patients what they needed, but never seemed to get ahead. Things just kept falling through the cracks.

"For example, everybody knew patients were supposed to get pneumonia vaccination shots. That seems like a little thing, but Medicare felt pneumonia vaccination was important enough to be a measure of a hospital's quality — they call it a Core Measure. So management exhorted us to do better. We tried to see that everybody got his or her vaccination. For a while it worked, and then we'd slip back. It was very difficult to sustain improvement.

"After starting Adaptive Design, we believed we *could* make a lasting difference. Management had us do a Focused Learning Event, where we take one problem — like pneumonia vaccination — and focus on testing improvements by problem solving as rapidly as possible. We started with our current protocol. Everybody thought it was 'best practice,' but in two weeks, we had improved it 12 times. Patients with vaccinations went from 65 percent to 100 percent. Now it is rare that someone doesn't get a vaccination — and, if we miss someone, we always pick it up and that just becomes another problem to solve, another opportunity to improve."

"Well, I can see how that makes a difference in patient care," Bill responded, "but it doesn't explain how I got my own parking place. Parking has always been a headache around here. You must have spent millions building new off-site parking for staff so that patients can park close to the door. And how'd you know A6 was my spot?"

Jane smiled again. "The learning was not limited to the nurses, doctors and managers. Everybody must identify problems — housekeepers, maintenance, central supply, the billing office. Even our parking valets. When you were here last year it took us six hours to deliver the 90 minutes of actual care you needed. The rest of the time was spent in waste, rework, redundancy and waiting.

"As we got better and better at small experiments to redesign the work, such waste, rework and redundancy started to go away. Even the waiting! Our teachers taught us that if you solve the small problems close to you, the big problems go too.

"Well, one of our biggest problems was parking. But, as patients and families spent less and less time waiting, our need for parking space started to decrease. This situation was uncovered by one of our parking valets who said, 'I have a problem because we are starting to have more parking spaces than we need, and patients still have to walk from the parking lots or wait for me to get their car. Can't we redesign our parking to be more Ideal for patients?'

"That one question led to a whole series of experiments around parking. You can't imagine what we learned. One reason that patients waited was because patients before them arrived late and knocked all of our schedules off. When we investigated the root cause, guess what? Many patients didn't know how to get here! That led to experimenting with sending every patient a map with estimated travel time. Getting the map off the Internet was a snap. Several more tests and we had a simple, reproducible, improvable system that the patients valued and helped us to become more efficient. Our 'late for admission' patients started to become fewer and fewer, and we got more accurate about the timing of our services.

"It was like a cycle of increasing returns: the more we worked on problem solving, the easier it got to be more efficient. We always thought we had to get the patients here early and have them wait so *we* wouldn't have to wait. What we found was that, not only was waiting less than Ideal for patients, it slowed everybody down. We had all grown to expect that everything would be late.

"Waiting had to go — and we knew it. Our teachers said we were becoming 'intolerant of mediocrity.' After many small experiments and also many little failures that helped us learn, we finally succeeded. About four months ago, we eliminated the last patient waiting room in outpatient surgery. And boy did we celebrate!

"Then, one day, another parking valet came up with the idea of the designated parking place. We were now so proficient at problem solving we knew when patients and their cars were here and also when they weren't. And that led to the test of designated parking for outpatients. Valets became parking coordinators and problem solvers who continually improved the system. Patients park themselves or use the valet — better, easier, quicker and closer than ever before."

This was a great story. But Ann was still puzzled. "How could management do all these projects and still get their regular work done? It seems impossible without hiring more managers."

Jane answered quickly. "That was another great discovery. Before Adaptive Design, everybody assumed management searched for answers while the rest of us did the work. We all discovered that Adaptive Design not only provided new skills and tools, the rules also created discipline, structure and consistency. Any problem that could be solved on the frontline should be solved there. Otherwise, management would get involved. Anything else is a waste of management time.

Next, we discovered we really needed management's broader vision to support and challenge us to pull this all together. In turn, management discovered their work needed to change. They needed to stop trying to solve all those big problems and increasingly support and challenge us to solve the little problems. It was a real change for everybody."

Bill and Ann were beginning to get the idea. St. TAH's management team had transitioned from being decision-makers who were separated from the work to developing, coordinating and controlling decision-rights that had been moved closer to the patient at the point-of-care.

Ann said, "I think I see now. So the Ideal Health Card was not bought from some computer vendor. You developed it yourselves."

"Exactly, Mrs. Jones. Nobody was happy with our old computer systems. Management bought state-of-the-art, but the systems were always over budget and under-performing — and a real headache for staff. I was spending more time looking at a computer screen and less time with my patients. Even the computer system became a problem to deal with.

"Management gave us the opportunity to test simple, inexpensive, new ideas. Their only requirements were to follow the Adaptive Design rules, use the same disciplined, structured, problem solving methods, and continue to move patient care toward Ideal. The necessary information was much simpler than anyone had imagined, and lots of inexpensive technologies were already available to do the job.

"Since outpatient surgery is the Learning Line, we were the first in the system to put the computer screens in the back office. Now, with your Ideal Health Card, this piece of paper and my PDA/cell phone, I have the information I need to still work with you and Mrs. Jones directly.

"But now I need to get you ready for your surgery, Mr. Jones. It's fun talking about all these things, but it's time to move to the operating room. Don't worry. I'll be with you back there also. Here's your hospital garb, and there is the locked closet. Mrs. Jones will have the key. I will be back in five minutes. Mrs. Jones can wait in the family and friends area. You and I are off to surgery."

Ann was pleasantly surprised by the family area. Staffed by a competent, well-trained volunteer, it was much larger than she had anticipated or first realized. She could now see that St. TAH had gained more necessary waiting room space by eliminating unnecessary waiting areas, such as patient reception. The space also had many privacy options and spaces for children to be quietly rambunctious. She also discovered another use for her Ideal Patient Card, when the volunteer showed her how to scan her location so she could be easily found.

Bill's operation went smoothly, and Jane RN was with him the whole way. Again, the personal nurse was not an implemented program, but rather the result of constant experimentation and learning. In their problem solving exercises the nursing staff had noticed that individual jobs were becoming simpler; as such, it became easier to cross-train for other positions.

Then one day, a nurse signaled a problem, "Why do I have to hand the patient off to another nurse to do admission, another to do pre-anesthesia, another in the operating room, another to the PACU, another to discharge? It is only one RN to one or two patients in many of those places. If we wanted to really simplify the work, couldn't one nurse follow a patient through without adding any additional staff?"

Again a flurry of small experiments had led to Jane's role. She and two other nurses were prototyping this personal nurse concept with Bill and several other patients that very day. A personal nurse actually required less nursing time per patient than the traditional system. It eliminated waiting for something to do and the need to report to others, just another example of obtaining more for less.

Bill had one more surprise, besides the fact that his surgery went well. With what he had seen and experienced, he expected as much. But while reconciling his Ideal Health Card just before discharge, Jane had surprisingly discovered that Bill had been given the wrong discharge medication. She signaled the problem by pressing a button by the door to their dressing room and another RN, Amy, entered. Jane explained the problem to Amy, her Learner/Leader/Teacher. Amy retrieved the correct medication, so Bill would not be delayed. Even more important, however, she would now seek an understanding not only of how the system had failed but also how it could be improved.

Bill knew they would find the solution and continue to relentlessly improve St. TAH. Both Bill and Ann knew where he would be having his surgery done next year. St. TAH's changes had made a difference.

And now, Scenario B: Bill's outpatient surgery experience at St. TAH's
if everyone had just continued to try harder. Bill's story...

Bill gets lost on the way to the hospital and arrives late. Then he has trouble finding parking, gets drenched in the rain and finds the waiting room full. Next he experiences multiple delays, many nurses and confusing transfers. Post-surgery, Bill experiences nausea, is discharged late and gets soaked again.

People want to help, but no one has the time, so no one but Bill notices or cares.

Is "Scenario A" a dream of the distant future? Not necessarily. Clinics, hospitals and health systems around the country are currently developing and using Adaptive Design. The key is not "what to do," but "how to do it."

If you're in any way involved in healthcare, Bill's story can become yours. But enough with stories. It's time for some straight talk!

CHAPTER 4

A DEMAND FOR CHANGE

"We can't solve problems by using the same kind
of thinking we used when we created them."

– ALBERT EINSTEIN

S ince you have picked up this book, you are probably involved in healthcare. As such, no one needs to tell you that today's healthcare environment is extremely complex. It's also dynamic and, more than anything else, it's unpredictable. Traditional methods for improvement have a high likelihood of failure. And yet change is not an option: it's a necessity.

For the past eight years, my colleagues and I have been working with hospitals and health systems across the country teaching the principles and practices of Adaptive Design.

I started by first researching disruptive, transformative innovation and then the driving force behind the success of the Toyota Production System (TPS), all the while asking, "Could these innovation and management secrets offer anything to healthcare?" After years of study, testing, learning and improving, one realization surfaced quite naturally: Toyota's success is not about manufacturing or managing processes. It's about people — how they work and manage, how they think about their work, how they learn and how together they improve.

These concepts lay the groundwork for Adaptive Design.

The Benefits of Adaptive Design

Adaptive Design works as an enabling technology that continually improves an organization's ability to deliver exactly what a patient needs while simultaneously lowering the cost of care. Viewing every employee as a valuable knowledge-worker, it revitalizes an organization so that each person becomes a skilled problem-solver. In the bigger picture, healthcare organizations trained in Adaptive Design have seen these great results:

- most improved patient satisfaction in an 17-hospital system,
- highest staff engagement scores for three years in a 12-hospital system,
- increased surgical volume by 16 percent while simultaneously decreasing surgical staff overtime by 14 percent and becoming 95 percent Joint Commission compliant, and
- self-sustaining local systems that increase productivity while simultaneously improving staff retention and recruitment.

Specifically, one Adaptive Design medical/surgical nursing unit showed a 51 percent decrease in staff turnover within one year while simultaneously improving financial performance by generating $1,700,000 in savings and new revenue in a 13-month period.

CEOs who incorporate Adaptive Design build a legacy of excellence. Employees in these transformed hospitals will have their energy and commitment restored, as jobs they previously wanted to escape turn into attractive and rejuvenating opportunities.

And, while quality is being improved, these same results show that healthcare costs are being lowered. There is no tradeoff!

However, while such results are inspiring and empowering, they are not enough reason for a medical facility to incorporate Adaptive Design.

Patient Care — the Primary Focus

The only valid consideration for adopting any innovation into your healthcare organization is this: *How will it affect patient care?*

Adaptive Design's primary focus is the patient. In fact, under this process the hospital becomes so patient-centered that adapting to meet patient needs is the natural, balanced, *default* response of everyone in the organization.

No One Can Stop Innovation, But...

Innovation *will* happen. For both good and bad, change is inevitable. With Adaptive Design, however, the frontline generates and management coordinates and challenges the innovation, providing structure while lowering the risks of change.

One visionary healthcare CEO confided this: "I know we have great ideas and are planning wonderful new innovations for our system. But what keeps me awake at night are my concerns that our people won't use them effectively. Will our employees change the ways they work to make use of the innovations? And will these innovations really make a difference?"

Innovation would be easier and less stressful if leaders could be sure that all changes were improvements. *And therein lies the rub.*

In my research, three factors make the difference between successful innovators and those that try hard, but don't succeed. Basically, it boils down to management's ability to:

1. make changes,
2. maximize the improvements that come from the changes, and
3. minimize any change-effects that are not improvements.

With apologies to a great and famous company, I call them the 3-Ms: *Make* changes. *Maximize* what works. *Minimize* what doesn't.

In one way or another, all great companies find a way to do the 3-Ms. What Toyota discovered is a disciplined, structured, reproducible way to accelerate the rate of change, maximize improvements and minimize the negative effects of change. Think of it as the 3-Ms — turbocharged. Capturing that same capability to *optimize* improvement is what sets Adaptive Design apart from other healthcare innovations!

Why Adaptive Design Works

For now, just assume that Adaptive Design works. In later chapters I will present the research and case studies. Some folks need "to see it to believe it." I'm waging that if you believe it, you will see it.

Adaptive Design succeeds because it is:

- a logical, direct extension of what you are currently doing — patient care — rather than some "radical" change,
- steady, progressive, sustainable growth — not a miracle or magic bullet,
- disciplined, structured, testable and verifiable — not a leap of faith,
- a rapid, measurable return on assets — not a big investment with an iffy long-term payoff, and
- "designed to adapt" — not last year's great idea based on last year's predictions.

A Commentary on the Future

The story in Chapter Three of patient Bill's experience with Jane RN at St. Typical American Hospital (St. TAH's) offers a forecast of the future. But how exaggerated was that picture?

Let's review the surprises Bill encountered. First, management, physicians and staff were working with a single-minded purpose — Ideal Patient Care — resulting in greater quality at less cost.

Next, Bill's experience with his reserved parking space was an initial pleasant surprise. His waiting time decreased by being assigned one personal nurse. Furthermore, the Ideal Health Card was efficient and time-saving. Overall, Bill experienced a self-reinforcing culture of effectiveness and safety, which alone diminishes a patient's stress.

This narrative only portrays what, in fact, people working in real healthcare organizations have been quietly learning and doing for years — under Adaptive Design.

Patients like Bill could not be more pleased!

What made the difference at St. TAH? Seven things:

1. Setting a clear direction made the difference!

Everyone on the St. TAH outpatient surgical unit was focused on one thing: Ideal Patient Care. Mission and values were important, but focusing on Ideal Patient Care became the way to achieve that mission and put those values to practice every day in productive, concrete and creative ways.

As you will see later in this book, Ideal Patient Care is an inspiring and aspiring real-time management tool.

Everyone knew where they were going.

2. Immediate, systemic problem solving made the difference!

Bill was concerned about errors and felt hassled by all the system failures he had encountered the previous year. St. TAH made a difference by identifying system failures as problems to be solved now. They made high performance and innovation part of everyone's daily work, with an operational framework disciplined and structured to solve a particular problem as near to the "snag" as possible.

Everyone became a problem solver, all the time.

3. Developing people — not things — made the difference!

Some folks believe that problem solving is about the problem. Adaptive Design would argue that it's more about the person working on the problem. Solving problems develops people. Every problem solved by Jane RN and her co-workers and/or managers increased their skills, confidence, trust and optimism.

Adaptive Design emphasizes personal attention. It is *people*, after all, who make the real difference. In our story Bill was able to connect with a *real person*, Jane RN, whose redesigned schedule made that connection possible.

In the past 38 years, I have seen administrative duties, information technology and the constant hassle of workarounds, tradeoffs and waiting progressively replace personal connections between patients and caregivers.

St. TAH's management reversed that trend by relentlessly eliminating administrative work and wasted time. That, in turn, created more time to focus on meeting patient needs — personally and directly.

Since *everyone counts, the focus is on developing people through problem solving, to meet patient needs Ideally.*

4. Simple "creative" technology made the difference!

In highly adaptive organizations (certainly Toyota is an example), technology is not "the big solution;" it is only *part* of the solution. It does a job.

Jim Collins, in his best-selling book, *Good to Great*, reports that almost never is it a big expensive technological product that moves an organization from good to great. Rather, as Collins says, small and cumulative "technological accelerators" are added over time to make a difference. But, again, they are just tools for the people who solve the problems.

For example, at this moment every hospital in America probably has access to all the simple technology needed to create, maintain and improve an Ideal Health Card. Such a card would be a technological accelerator for registration, increased safety *and* a platform for new business growth.

Technology is not magic; it just does a job. And why buy it when you can make it?

5. All together, problem solving + people + simple technology made the difference!

As Jane explained to Bill, the changes at St. TAH did not happen from a one-time design implementation. Instead, improvements were made and remade daily. A common strategic purpose focused with clarity and consistency empowered the knowledge, creativity and problem solving abilities of people — 7 days a week, 365 days a year.

Every employee in the outpatient surgery unit was accountable to each other for making inquiry and core business execution part of his or her daily work.

6. By relentlessly challenging what employees had already learned and always believed, cycles of increasing returns were created that made the difference!

Everyone at Toyota focuses on the return on assets (ROA), and management is relentless in its efforts to challenge each employee to improve at every opportunity.

St. TAH's management team taught the *value* of ROA, demonstrated the benefits of challenging and improving, and provided the rules and support that made it all possible.

Instead of exhorting everyone to "try harder," St. TAH's management rekindled the latent energy and desire to improve that lies in the heart of almost everyone in healthcare. The first step down the Adaptive Design path leads to results that make a difference. And the more it's done, the better it gets, creating cycles of increasing returns. The energy is contagious. Bill recognized it immediately when he walked through the door.

The "waits, delays, unanticipated results, obscure instructions and harried people rushing from place to place" that Bill had previously experienced became problems solved. Ambiguity, assumptions, workarounds and tradeoffs were eliminated, all as a result of Adaptive Design.

The experience of structured problem solving molded staff, physician and management attitudes and enhanced their abilities. And quick results reinforced the learning. Like flushing out small grains of sand grinding away in the wheels and gears of the system for years, patient care and safety were improved, waiting times decreased and outpatient surgery services transformed. Then, by lowering the number of patients waiting, fewer cars remained in the previously overcrowded parking lot.

No surprise, however, since all machine parts run smoother when the gears are progressively cleaned.

Soon the "buzz" spread that St. TAH was different. This led to increased patient volume. More volume — at lower cost — means higher profit and the option to *decrease* the cost of care.

Higher quality at lower cost and improved patient care — those are the guideposts along the Adaptive Design path and a formula for success that creates hope for patients, nurtures morale among staff, and leaves a legacy of accomplishment and success for leadership.

Management focused on developing people — not processes or things.

7. Acting your way to a new way of thinking makes the difference!

A common saying at Toyota is, "You cannot know until you see. You cannot see until you do." Current management procedures and methods (based on the traditional industrial model) have people thinking their way to a new way of acting. In highly innovative companies, however, acting your way to a new way of thinking is the norm. *Adaptive Design proves acting your way to a new way of thinking makes a difference in healthcare too!*

The next chapter describes disruptive innovation — what happens when the inability to adapt to a changing environment disrupts established organizations and institutions. Using a medical metaphor, disruptive innovation is a complex but reliable *symptom* that signals the need for an organization to adapt and change.

Disruption is happening in healthcare now!

How good is your organization at handling adaptation and change? The path is clear. The time for change is now. You might be the next innovator to become *designed to adapt.*

CHAPTER 5

DISRUPTIVE INNOVATION: TO STOP THE MACHINE

"To see, to hear, means nothing.
To recognize (or not to recognize) means everything..."

– André Breton

B reton's quote defines my first-year experience at Harvard's Kennedy School in 1997, where my goals certainly were "to see, to hear." Not long into the program, however, I learned that "to recognize or not to recognize" was the part of the equation that mattered most.

From first-hand experience as both a patient and physician, I knew that business-as-usual in healthcare was not working. I sought answers on what it would take to create an environment that both honored and nurtured new ideas. Could the radical innovations necessary to "fix" healthcare happen even in an established setting?

Answers directly from research were unexpected: Leading companies find it very difficult to *recognize* certain kinds of new opportunities and almost *never* recognize certain kinds of threats.

Clayton M. Christensen, Professor at Harvard Business School, taught me how to recognize the differences between opportunities and threats.

Prior to his book, *The Innovator's Dilemma*, change was expected to come from industry leaders. His theory of disruptive innovation stretched my brain to a new place.

Who better to build the new mousetrap than those with resources and mousetrap know-how? Yet, in his study of over 300 companies and industries, Christensen concluded that, more often than not, transformational innovation emerges from far outside the established hierarchy. In other words, when an entire industry is undergoing transformation, the better known "top" companies typically are *not* the transformational innovators.

The following table illustrates this concept: The left shows established leaders, the right, "disruptive innovators."

Table I	
Leaders and Innovators	
THE ESTABLISHED LEADERS	THE DISRUPTIVE INNOVATORS
Digital Equipment Company	Microsoft, Apple, IBM
Macy's, Marshall Field's, Sears	Nordstrom, Target, Wal-Mart
GM, Ford, Chrysler	Toyota
Merrill Lynch, Lehman Brothers	Charles Schwab, Vanguard
United, American, Delta	Southwest Airlines
Microsoft	Google

Christensen's research shows that often a company's best qualities lie at the root of its failure to innovate. "Great capabilities," he writes, "can also be disabilities." Most organizations excel in what they are designed to do. Typically, management decides what works, then resolves to repeat and improve it. The greatest organizations excel at this formula: repeat and improve.

Let me emphasize this point: High performance companies focus on optimizing and improving what they do successfully. While usually the improvements are incremental, they could also be highly creative breakthroughs, leading to new businesses that benefit humankind, empower the company and increase profitability. Business journals continue to document the inspiring stories.

So, why is total transformation difficult, if not nearly impossible?

Here's the problem: Successful, traditionally managed companies are not designed to *reinvent the wheel*. They need economies of scale based on what works for them, i.e., their own "wheel." They want to optimize what works, not what fails. As such, they establish organizational DNA — structures, processes, technology — that can only advance and improve their own wheel. And they hire and carefully train people to perpetuate the habits, behaviors and values that keep that wheel turning! How far are you going to get in your organization by saying, "I want to optimize what we fail at doing." That's not the way to the top in most companies.

Therefore, success is deeply imbedded in the DNA of high performance companies — which is the problem! The successful organization's DNA works well until somebody comes up with a "new wheel" — a new business model (DNA) based on more accessible and less costly products or services that meet new customer demands. Just as it is almost impossible for an organism to change its DNA, it's almost impossible for that leading organization to change.

For example, no airline challenged the leaders, like American, United and Delta — *until* Southwest. General Motors dominated car manufacturing for decades — *until* Toyota. Since then, American, United, Delta and GM have found it almost impossible to compete.

"Men at some time are masters of their fates: The fault, dear Brutus, is not in our stars, but in ourselves," penned Shakespeare, in *Julius Caesar*. Christensen showed that the very qualities that help companies rise to success can become barriers that can't be overcome by merely "trying harder." In those circumstances, it's not what you do that counts: *it's what you do when you don't know what to do that really makes the difference*! Adaptive Design enables leadership to find solutions when current structures and methods have become part of the problem.

When a new business unseats the best-of-the-best, Christensen calls this *disruptive innovation* — a transformation that established organizations find almost *impossible* to duplicate or compete against. In his article "Disruptive Innovation for Social Change," published in the *Harvard Business Review* (December, 2006), Christensen writes:

> The existing players in any sector have resources, processes, partners, and business models designed to support the status quo. This makes it difficult and unappealing for them to challenge the prevailing way of doing things. Organizations are set up to support their existing business models...[I]t is almost impossible for them to disrupt themselves.

As I present Christensen's work in healthcare settings, I often hear the comment: "Very interesting. But it doesn't apply to us. Disruptive innovation does not occur in healthcare."

The essence of disruptive innovation is that a simple concept or technology, ignored by the leading institutions, creates a fundamentally improved way to work.

Take a look at Table 2. Then tell me if disruptive innovation has, or has not, made a difference in healthcare.

Table 2 Disruptive Innovation in Healthcare		
THE BEGINNING?	SIMPLE CONCEPT/ TECHNOLOGY?	THE RESULT?
An outcast Austrian MD frustrated by epidemic obstetric infections	Semmelweis' germ theory of infection and insistence on sanitary birth conditions	The concepts of sterility, antisepsis and antibiotics
Care of poor pregnant women in 1840s Boston	Multi-disciplinary obstetric services to the poor	Brigham and Women's Hospital; Boston, MA
Two dissatisfied brother surgeons in a small, mid-western town	"There is no place for individuality in healthcare"	Mayo Clinic and the concept of the employed MD multi-specialty clinic
Recruiting Depression-Era Dallas school teachers	Employer-paid healthcare insurance	Blue Cross/Blue Shield
WW II shipyard workers with no healthcare in Vancouver, WA	Prepaid healthcare and employed physicians	Kaiser Permanente
Portland, OR radiologist dilating arteries with rubber catheters	Direct mechanical dilatation of atherosclerotic arteries	Cardiac and peripheral arterial angioplasty

I found Christensen's work not only informative — but inspiring!

And he found *my* vision challenging. Christensen's interest in developing the theory of disruptive innovation for healthcare led to my invitation to become a Visiting Scholar at Harvard Business School. That created the opportunity to learn more about disruptive innovation and begin to develop the concept for healthcare. Christensen, Jerome Grossman, MD, and Jason Hwang, MD, subsequently greatly expanded that germ of an idea and their book, *The Innovator's Prescription*, is the "Bible" on the disruption of healthcare.

With Christensen's lead, rather than focusing only on healthcare-related businesses, I was also inspired to investigate non-healthcare organizations. At Harvard Business School I was like a kid in a candy story — and the candy I eventually discovered was Toyota.

Christensen's work shows that established companies usually never transform their own industries. It's as though they have a "blind spot" when it comes to transformational, disruptive innovation. In fact, the more successful the company, the harder it is for that organization to transform

— even if failing to do so could lead to its demise. Sadly, history suggests that established organizations may be perfectly designed for failure!

So how can an organization use (rather than suppress) humankind's natural ability to adapt?

The answer came by first examining startups that became successful disruptive innovators, e.g., Southwest Airlines and Microsoft.

Then I studied the few *established* companies that Christensen identified who defied the rules and were able to disrupt themselves, such as Intel, who under Andy Grove, twice disrupted itself; Hewlett-Packard's disruptive ink jet printers; IBM's disruptive personal computers; and Dayton-Hudson department stores that disruptively transformed into Target.

Finally, I studied Toyota and found there a company that creates great new businesses by continually breaking the rules. Toyota is an established organization that *disruptively transforms* itself in ways hard to duplicate.

All these different companies share certain common traits, which I have turned into principles. If applied correctly, these principles harness the natural, creative adaptability of humans and channel it to meet a company's innovation needs. Furthermore, these principles work with documented success for even the most complex business in America: healthcare.

Changing an organization also means changing its culture. One fundamental challenge faced by organizations desiring to become disruptive innovators is that it turns the old-style industrial model on its head with a unique way of looking at work performance, decision-making and management techniques. While that might seem intimidating, it actually is not a radical concept.

Most innovation has its origins at the grass-roots level and is born out of a deep understanding of how something works. In biology, *adaptation* is defined as "an alteration or adjustment in structure or habits by which a species or individual improves its condition in relationship to the environment." As such, an adaptive organization *embraces* change as an opportunity.

Clearly, adapting can be hard work. Christensen says that it's almost impossible for an established organization to transform itself. But *almost impossible* means something *is* possible. The concept of Adaptive Design grew from my desire to "expand the possible" for healthcare.

Expanding the possible for healthcare is my mission — and Adaptive Design is the method! But any transformation, even one built on simple principles, is not easy. Therefore, knowing if your organization needs to transform is an important first question.

This self-assessment, based on your experience, will tell you (1) if your institution needs to change, and (2) to what extent it may be vulnerable to competition, either from major rivals or disruptive innovators currently "under the radar."

The Hospital / Health System Self-Assessment Test

Based on your personal experience, answer the following questions yes or no.

COMPETITION	YES	NO
1. Is loss of profitable services or products one of your organization's top business issues?		
2. Is your organization facing competition that gains advantage by "not playing on a level field," e.g., cherry-picking simple or the most lucrative businesses?		
3. Are competitors fragmenting previously stable services or products?		
4. Are previously loyal physician groups and/or former business partners starting or threatening to compete against your organization?		
5. Has your organization used mergers and acquisitions to increase market power or consolidate to take capacity out of the market place?		
COST	YES	NO
6. Is decreasing costs one of your organization's top business issues?		
7. Is decreasing the cost of employees one of your top cost-control issues?		
8. Has your organization engaged in a restructuring or downsizing in the last twenty-four months?		
9. Do previously successful business lines now face elimination because of decreasing profitability?		
OPERATIONS	YES	NO
10. Are benchmarking and implementing better operational metrics top management issues?		
11. Is declining employee engagement one of your top management issues?		
12. Is improving patient satisfaction one of your top management issues?		
13. Is PDCA, 6 Sigma, Lean, Lean/Sigma or other process improvement methodologies one of your top management issues?		
14. Is finding and implementing more best practices one of your top management issues?		
15. Is your organization making increasingly large investments in information technology, facilities and other capital-intensive solutions?		
16. Is your organization focused increasingly on legislative initiatives, regulatory issues, and/or new sources of governmental and non-governmental funding?		
IN GENERAL	YES	NO
17. Do you believe healthcare needs to transform?		
18. Has your personal job satisfaction diminished over the last ten years?		

Questions 1-16, Score FIVE for Yes and ZERO for No.
Questions 17-18, Score TEN for Yes and ZERO for No. Highest possible score = 100.

The Key:

Score 0 – 30 — You have an unusually successful adaptive healthcare organization. If you are a multipurpose hospital, please give me a call. You can teach us all something!

Score 31 – 60 — You are pushing the end of your current business model. You probably face disruptive competitors. Trying harder at what you currently know how to do is not the answer. There's time, but you need to start to learn to adapt.

Score 61 – 100 — Things may seem okay. Yours may be a great leading institution. But you are tightening down the screws on your current business model. You gain temporary relief, then have to tighten some more. The tighter it gets, the more it hurts. You are probably beginning to experience recurrent cycles of profit and loss. If you are still profitable, you must invest in adaptive change. If you are struggling, you still have a chance to escape. But you must begin to adapt now.

Disruptive innovation shows that the efforts of successful companies stall unless strategies, tactics, systems or organizational structures change to meet altered conditions of competition. This includes the habits, behaviors and values of people working in those structures and systems.

American-born Lady Nancy Astor, the first woman to serve as a member of the British Parliament, made this observation: "The main dangers in this life are the people who want to change everything — or nothing." Her wisdom cannot be overemphasized.

The key, as I will show in subsequent chapters, is not to change everything, *but to be sure to change something*. Then learn and change some more.

Unfortunately, change is usually born of necessity. As such, disruptive innovation can be the very distraction an organization needs most, because it provides the framework and language for transformation. Christensen's data, combined with my experience, has led me to promulgate three laws for governing transformational innovation in established companies:

1. **Trying harder is not the answer.** The faster the rate of change in your industry, the more it becomes true that what you are currently doing *will not* be the source of your future success. Rather, the difference

is how effectively you adapt what you are currently doing to a constantly changing world.

2. **The "DNA" embedded in high performing organizations will always seek to slow, stall or stop adaptive change.** Don't feel guilty about it; it's a Law of Nature.

3. **Organizations "designed to adapt" will have the competitive advantage.** In the field of healthcare, they will define the future!

So, what exactly does "designed to adapt" look like? Chapter 6 will provide the rules and guidelines for Adaptive Design's amazing ability to build adaptive capacity into the daily work of everyone in the organization. The rules become the DNA.

ADAPTIVE DESIGN IN PRACTICE: THE RULES-IN-USE

"When... rules of life are taken away, the loss cannot possibly be estimated. From that moment, we have no compass to govern us, nor can we know distinctly to what port to steer."

– EDMUND BURKE

More books have been written about Toyota than about any other organization, and perhaps no company's methods have been more carefully studied by management scientists. Almost every author and business scholar has looked at Toyota through the lens of the Industrial or Process Management Model. Their findings show that *standardized* work is not only commonplace in Toyota, it's almost a religion.

As such, to emulate Toyota's results, an organization would have to emulate their methods and identify best practices. That only makes sense. But what are the *real* best practices at Toyota?

Not until 1999 did two scholars from the Harvard Business School articulate in simple terms Toyota's unique approach to management. The researchers were Harvard Business School Professors Steven Spear and H. Kent Bowen. It was my fortunate opportunity to work with and learn from Spear and Bowen as their ideas were maturing that led to testing these concepts in healthcare and, ultimately, Adaptive Design.

In retrospect, both Toyota's methods and insights seem obvious, as so often the case with inspired thought. The differences are amplified when you take off the lens of the traditional industrial process model and look at Toyota as an adaptive knowledge management company. But in the 1990's it was not clear at all. And it took years of study and work for Spear and Bowen to crack the code and identify and codify the four unwritten rules that govern the way people manage, learn and work at Toyota — individually and collectively.

In Adaptive Design, these rules become the framework and common language for learning, understanding and improving the work of healthcare.

The four "Rules-In-Use" (see Figure 1, next page) were first outlined in "Decoding the DNA of the Toyota Production System" (Spear & Bowen, *Harvard Business Review*, 1999, 95 - 106). This article documents a masterpiece of research and its concepts were key to the development of Adaptive Design.

Spear and Bowen studied over 40 different plants, some that used the Toyota Production System (TPS) and some that did not. Their investigative methods were unique: Spear went to work at the companies. After four years of hard work, diligent study, observation, and experience, the researchers were able to better understand the work of Toyota (an extremely complex organization) and define it in a simple, Toyota-like way with the four Rules-In-Use. The four rules combine three elements of work with one method of work improvement and problem solving. First, let's examine the three work elements:

1. **Activities** — the work of an individual, unaided. (Or, several people with a short-term common outcome to achieve.)
2. **Connections** — the simplest of teams: two people. (Since one person can't do it all, how do two people link to complete tasks?)
3. **Pathways** — complex teams of people and resources. ("Pathways" are how many people, supplies, equipment and technologies interconnect to produce complex goods or services.)

In Chapter 7 we will explore the fourth and final rule, showing how the work is improved through problem solving.

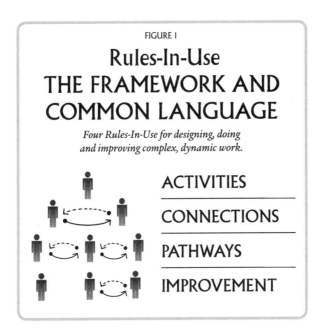

FIGURE 1

Rules-In-Use
THE FRAMEWORK AND
COMMON LANGUAGE

*Four Rules-In-Use for designing, doing
and improving complex, dynamic work.*

ACTIVITIES

CONNECTIONS

PATHWAYS

IMPROVEMENT

Rule 1: Activities are highly specified as to content, sequence, timing and outcome.

The first rule describes how an individual works within the Toyota Production System (TPS) and how design governs activity:

- *Content* refers to the steps of the work process.
- *Sequence* refers to the order in which the steps are performed.
- *Timing* refers to the amount of time required for each step.
- *Outcome* refers to the expected result from performing each sequential step in the work process.

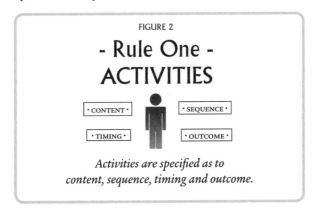

FIGURE 2

- Rule One -
ACTIVITIES

· CONTENT ·   · SEQUENCE ·

· TIMING ·   · OUTCOME ·

*Activities are specified as to
content, sequence, timing and outcome.*

45

Spear and Bowen explain that when a Toyota worker installs a car seat in a Toyota assembly plant, the work is specified so that the bolts are always tightened in the same order, each bolt turned in the same amount of time, and the torque to which the bolt should be tightened specified exactly.

The authors note that this level of exactness applies to repetitive motions of production workers and also to the activities of *all* employees in the organization. The rules are valid from the frontline worker to the CEO, so that everyone at Toyota is working off the same page.

First, let's look at this unique approach with a factory floor example.

In analyzing how seat installation is done outside of Toyota, Spear and Bowen found that at companies not practicing the Toyota Production System, the worker was expected to "take four bolts from a cardboard box, carry them and a torque wrench to the car, tighten the four bolts, then enter a code into a computer to indicate that the work had been done without problems." New workers were usually trained by an experienced colleague, who might be available to help the inexperienced person with any difficulties encountered, such as failing to tighten the bolt sufficiently or forgetting to enter the computer code.

So what's the problem with this non-TPS approach? Spear and Bowen point out that such an approach allows (in fact, *assumes*) considerable variation in the way employees do their work. We might say that they have "flexibility."

The problem with flexibility is that there is a great deal of opportunity for the new worker to install the seat differently than an experienced operator. Such variation could translate to poorer quality or better quality, by either the new employee or the experienced worker. But how would anyone know which way is better?

More importantly, variable work "hinders learning and improvement in the organization because the variations hide the link between how the work is done and the results," say Spear and Bowen.

In the adaptive knowledge management model, this is the single most important fact about work specificity: *If you know exactly how a job is done, and you know precisely when it fails, you now have a clear set of benchmarks against which to measure possible improvements.*

At Toyota, *it's not the process that is important, it is the learning.* This type of thinking exemplifies the vast difference between traditional industrial process management approaches and adaptive knowledge management at Toyota:

- Traditional management and process improvement methodologies seek to create uniformity by identifying best practices,[8] standardizing and implementing them, and then holding workers in alignment and accountable to perform them.
- Toyota's adaptive knowledge management approach standardizes work locally, *so it is easy to know when and how to change.*

Standardize — not to create uniformity, but to enable change! How can that be? Toyota management believes it cannot design perfect processes. Even "perfect designs" eventually fail, because the local environment will change in unknown and unknowable ways.

Therefore, Toyota has very few "industry standard best practices" for specific work. Instead, the management of each production facility focuses on learning as quickly as possible when a local process fails so that it can be improved as rapidly as possible.

Creating standard work locally makes it easier to identify a failing process and quickly design an improvement. Therefore, standard work in one Toyota plant may be very different than standard work for a similar job in another plant. *Standardization is a tool to facilitate change, not uniformity.*

In healthcare, work is currently standardized around best practices, with the goal of creating widespread uniformity and accountability. When the work varies, leaders can get it back into alignment with the standard. That's the traditional, industrial process management approach.

But Toyota does not work that way. Toyota standardizes locally to facilitate improvement and customize to local conditions. It can then identify when current methods change or fail, and gauge the results as quickly and simply as possible.

It is the 3-Ms again that I mentioned in Chapter 4: **make** change, **maximize** change that is an improvement, **minimize** change that is not. (Chapter 7 will show you how to use Rule 4, the improvement rule, to transform standardization from rigid uniformity to flexible responsiveness. For now, we will explore examples of the Rules-In-Use in real-life, real-time healthcare.)

Rule 1 then provides the framework that makes activities testable, verifiable and improvable. Here is a healthcare example using Rule 1, applicable to any large organization.

---

8 Best practices can be an ambiguous, confusing term, particularly when approaching work in Adaptive Design. See best practices in the Glossary for more clarity.

Healthcare Meetings Designed as Rule 1: Activities

The next time you are responsible for a meeting, instead of creating a standard agenda, test the power of Rule 1. Start first by identifying the desired *Outcome*, i.e., where you want the group to be when the meeting ends. Then, specify the *Content* (the specific points you need to include), the *Sequence* (the order in which those points will be addressed), and the *Timing* (the time taken for each point to be addressed).

During the actual meeting, if you fall behind the specified Timing, you know immediately you will have a problem achieving your Outcome without some adjustment. At the end of a meeting, always leave time for the test: *Did we achieve our stated Outcome?* If the answer is "Yes," you have completed the work as designed. If it is "No," then you have a problem to solve.

As you become more practiced in applying Adaptive Design to meetings, you may decide to start by specifying the Outcome and then have the group quickly create and improve the Content, Sequence, and Timing. In this way, you will engage everyone's knowledge and creativity towards achieving the desired Outcome. With the test at the end, everyone will own the result, and you will be managing knowledge.

One CEO uses Rule 1 to design all her senior leadership team and board meetings, specified as Activities. As such, all her meetings have clear, testable outcomes and built-in feedback, easy to adjust if the meeting's course goes astray from the initial design. She exemplifies Adaptive Design by practicing Adaptive Design!

If one person could do everything in healthcare, Rule 1 would be all that was needed. But healthcare is much too complex, dynamic and unpredictable for one person. Many varied connections to other people, supplies and technology are needed to meet patient needs Ideally. This takes us to Rule 2: Connections.

Rule 2: Connections.

Rule 2 directly addresses information and material transfer between individuals by governing how people connect with each other.

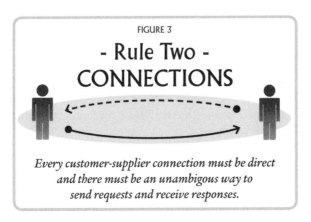

FIGURE 3

- Rule Two -
CONNECTIONS

Every customer-supplier connection must be direct and there must be an unambigous way to send requests and receive responses.

Here are the elements of Rule 2, as described by Spear and Bowen: Every connection must be standardized and direct. And every connection must unambiguously specify;

- the people involved,
- the form and quantity of the goods and/or services provided,
- the way requests are made, and
- the expected time in which the requests will be met.

This rule establishes a "customer-supplier" relationship between each worker and the person responsible for providing that individual with a specific good or service. "As a result, there are no gray zones in deciding who provides what to whom and when," according to Spear and Bowen.

Through the viewfinder of Rule 2, let's look at a typical healthcare connection. How does a surgeon obtain the instruments needed during an operation? (While this example may seem trivial, *it is applicable to anyone being supplied equipment or information anywhere* in the institution. Learn by doing. Test it yourself and see.)

Following Rule 2, first specify the people involved:

- The customer is the surgeon.
- The supplier is the surgical scrub technician.

How does the supplier know what to supply? Rule 2 states that the "form and quantity must be unambiguously specified."

Under Adaptive Design, the customer is obligated to first define exactly what he or she needs. Therefore, the surgeon must know and then announce! For example, if she wants two types of scissors during the operation (dissecting scissors and suture scissors), specifying that ahead of time is the surgeon's responsibility. Having it available is the supplier scrub tech's responsibility.

Next, the customer and supplier must specify and agree on how requests are to be made. In Adaptive Design, customers always initiate the request; it is not up to the supplier to guess what and when to deliver. Toyota refers to this as a "pull system:" the customer pulls the supplier by signaling in a specified way, "I need X."

In this case, the surgeon says, "Suture scissors," and holds out her hand. The surgical technician supplies the scissors by placing them in the surgeon's hand in a specified way within a specified time, e.g., two to three seconds. An illustration of this connection might look like Figure 4:

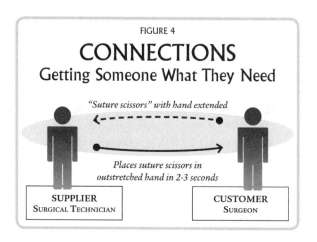

FIGURE 4

CONNECTIONS
Getting Someone What They Need

"Suture scissors" with hand extended

Places suture scissors in outstretched hand in 2-3 seconds

SUPPLIER
Surgical Technician

CUSTOMER
Surgeon

Any failure in this connection can then be immediately identified as a problem to be solved — no ambiguity, no assumptions.

While not rocket science, this is much different from many traditional operating room practices where the specifics are left vague, ill-defined, and therefore, unable to be improved. For example, in many operating rooms, the standard practice is that the tech is expected to anticipate the surgeon's needs. In an Adaptive Design OR, the exact needs are specified by the customer-surgeon.

Common to nearly all complex work is the coordination of people and activities — from building homes to performing open-heart surgery. But in most instances, "customer-supplier" relationships are ambiguous and unspecified. Unspecified connections, ubiquitous in healthcare, are the source of many problems.

For example, any supervisor can usually answer a call for help. That sounds efficient and "flexible." Yet, as Spear and Bowen point out, the difficulty with such an approach is that "when something is everybody's problem, it becomes no one's problem."

If two people could do everything in healthcare, Rule 1 and specified connections as Rule 2 would be all we would have to consider. But healthcare is much more complicated. Many people, technologies, supplies and much equipment must come together in a coordinated way to create a complex service. That requires another Rule.

Rule 3: Pathways.

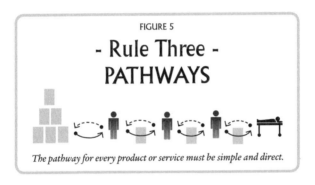

FIGURE 5

- Rule Three -
PATHWAYS

The pathway for every product or service must be simple and direct.

The focus of Rule 2 is the customer-supplier relationship. The focus of Rule 3 is to link these connections: "The pathway for every product and service must be simple and direct."

Linking many customer-supplier connections creates pathways over which to develop complex goods or services. An important starting point is to clearly identify who is — or is not — included in a Rule 3 pathway. Every necessary person and/or technology "supplier" is included; unnecessary persons or technologies are not included.

Harvard Business School researchers Anita Tucker and Amy Edmondson, observed that "the unpredictable nature of healthcare and the high level of interdependence among service-providing employees (e.g., nurses, doctors, pharmacy, central supply, and laboratory) make it likely that nurses will encounter failures in the course of their day-to-day work." Pathways in healthcare can be convoluted and unspecific, causing problems that lead to system failures. Research shows that these failures are likely to be the result of problems resulting from faulty "customer-supplier" connections (Rule 2) or problems along the complex pathways where supplies and services move in the healthcare setting (Rule 3).

Toyota illustrates pathways in drawings they call "Material and Information Flows" (M&I Flow). Figure 6 shows the first M&I Flow done in healthcare — a drawing I made of medication delivery (let's say an Aspirin tablet) on a unit in one of America's Top-Ten Hospitals.

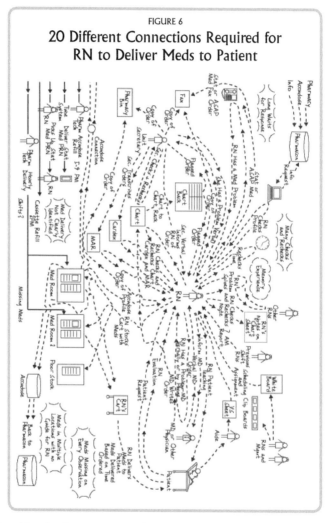

FIGURE 6
20 Different Connections Required for RN to Deliver Meds to Patient

Consider the dynamic, unpredictable complexity represented here. Such complexity is typical of every hospital we have studied. And, in our experience, imposing a new computer system on top of this turbulent flow is not the solution.

Returning to our surgeon and surgical technician example, let's look at how Toyota would approach the pathway problem of a surgeon getting her suture scissors exactly when needed.

Toyota discovered many years ago that it is much easier to represent pathways and connections in drawings. (Our Adaptive Design experience in healthcare has confirmed that approach.) Figure 7 shows a hypothetical pathway for supplying suture scissors to a surgeon during her procedure. You can use these same conventions to decipher the Aspirin example in Figure 6.

- Dotted lines represent "Information." Information in Toyota's adaptive knowledge management system has a very specific function: It tells you what to do to deliver the customer's needs "Ideally." (Note: In almost all healthcare pathways the end customer is the patient.)
- Solid lines represent the flow of materials or services back to the end customer.
- People are stick figures.
- All the other points along the pathway are drawn where they belong in the customer-supplier relationship, not geographically in the hospital. In this case, the preference card, inventory, instrument kit and the scrub tech's OR table are all drawn where they fit on the pathway.
- Start with the patient on the right and work back following the information counterclockwise along the pathway to inventory, then back to the patient with the appropriate supplies.

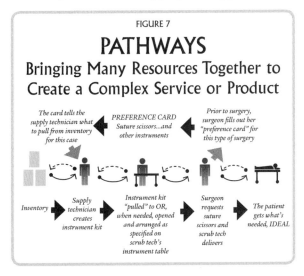

FIGURE 7

PATHWAYS
Bringing Many Resources Together to Create a Complex Service or Product

The card tells the supply technician what to pull from inventory for this case

PREFERENCE CARD
Suture scissors...and other instruments

Prior to surgery, surgeon fills out her "preference card" for this type of surgery

Inventory

Supply technician creates instrument kit

Instrument kit "pulled" to OR, when needed, opened and arranged as specified on scrub tech's instrument table

Surgeon requests suture scissors and scrub tech delivers

The patient gets what's needed, IDEAL

The following presents a verbal description of the M&I Flow that supplies scissors to the surgeon just when she needs it. (Note: It does not represent a "Best Practice" or the final solution for all surgical supply problems.) This is a hypothetical example of what might happen in an operating room, illustrating the concept of Rule 3 "Pathways" and M&I Flow.

1. The surgeon is accountable to know what she needs and to fill out a "preference card" that will describe all the instruments (including the "suture scissors") needed for each type of surgery performed.
2. The information on this card is then "pulled" by the supply technician at a specified time prior to surgery.
3. The surgical technician takes this information at a specified time to the surgical instrument inventory to assemble all the instruments needed for this case.
4. The instruments are transported to the operating room as an "instrument kit," specific to this surgery when called for ("pulled") by the surgical tech.
5. The instrument kit is first sterilized and then opened and distributed by a surgical scrub tech on the instrument table in the operating room at a specified time and arranged in a specified way.
6. When the surgeon discovers she needs a suture scissors to meet the patient's needs during this specific surgery, she completes the connection as specified (see Rule 2, page 48) above.

Many readers familiar with the operating room might say, "So what! We've used preference cards for years. There is nothing new here. Where's the computerized system that Toyota uses to manage the logistics of highly variable part distribution?"

The answer is obvious only if you look at Toyota through the lens of an adaptive knowledge management model: The "computers" in this analogy are the minds of the people doing this work; the "software" are Rules-In-Use. The "who" is the people doing the work — those best able to solve problems in the system when it fails. And fail it will. There is nothing magic about preference cards or computerized OR supply systems.

In my 35 years as a surgeon, I have never found a general hospital operating room — with or without computers — that could reliably deliver instruments on time and as needed.

Adaptive Design explains why. Complex, unpredictable changes constantly happen at every point of the M&I Flow diagram. What we *can* predict is that unknown problems will affect this pathway and will cause failures.

In a typical hospital, those failures are simply more aggravating problems to be solved in an *ad hoc*, haphazard way or "fixed" with a rigid, "standardized," top-down approach. In an Adaptive Design hospital, those failures become opportunities for improvement.

How then do we fix these system failures? What happens when the surgeon fails to fill out her preference card or decides to add a new instrument? What happens when the preference card fails to deliver what's needed? How do you get people to do what they are supposed to do?

Adaptive Design redefines system failures as "problems to be solved." The next chapter details the method. But before we go there, let's again examine both accountability and problems.

Is it people or systems that create accountability?

Healthcare often relies on individual experience, intelligence and diligence to improve work processes. This extremely personal approach towards improvement relies on individual recognition of failed techniques and outcomes, as well as *ad hoc* learning about ways to improve. Fortunately, the healthcare workforce is generally both intelligent and diligent. The problem with this approach is the inevitable wide variation in experience among healthcare workers.

Have you ever had the awkward experience of having blood drawn by a physician who performs such tasks infrequently? Now compare that experience to having blood drawn by an experienced phlebotomist. In which case is the work likely to be most highly specified in terms of "content, sequence, timing and outcome?" Who is likely to achieve the best outcome?

And, most importantly, whose work is easiest to improve? As Spear and Bowen point out, a better outcome is only one facet of why work specificity is important. Without such specificity, it is difficult to know how or when things go wrong and hard to understand where and how to improve them when they do.

The phlebotomist, who through trial and error has specified her work, is much more likely to identify problems, evaluate changes and improve. But rather than leave this improvement up to the diligence of an individual, at Toyota and in Adaptive Design, problem solving and improvement are rule-based and part of the "system." The high level of specificity and sensitivity to problems that enables people to engage in a rigorous and continuous process of testing and improvement is the basis for Toyota's adaptive knowledge management model and is the essence of Adaptive Design in healthcare.

This improvement-based problem solving starts with a detailed assessment of the current state of affairs, then goes on to institute a plan for improvement that is essentially an experimental test of proposed changes.

Providing highly specialized patient care is far different from assembling automobiles. In healthcare, standardization (especially with respect to the content, sequence and timing of activities) is challenging. For example, routine nursing care to a frail 78-year-old woman with lung disease will vary from a more mobile and alert 65-year-old cancer patient. The daily care each patient receives will almost certainly be unpredictable beyond a very short timeframe. Therefore, the use of Adaptive Design at the point-of-care mandates that each patient's treatment must be equally appropriate, locally standardized, updated and improved as conditions change.

In reality, this is what great nursing has truly been about since its beginnings — highly individualized care, continually customized to meet the patient's constantly changing needs. Toyota's adaptive knowledge management methods and Adaptive Design both verify that the higher the degree of complexity, the more important it is for the frontline to specify work, then identify problems and solve them systematically. The first step is to identify problems as *opportunities*.

So, let's look again at problems in healthcare, starting with an attitude not heard often in corporate settings: **"Thank goodness, we've failed and found a problem."**

Admitting that problems will typically arise in healthcare, let's revisit the surprising research findings of Tucker and Edmondson I introduced in Chapter 1. Their article, "Why Hospitals Don't Learn From Failure: Organizational and Psychological Dynamics that Inhibit System Change," describes some unrecognized problems inherent in the current system, along with insight into how Toyota's rules that govern conduct actually accelerate learning and work improvement.

Tucker and Edmondson, investigating how nurses responded to failures in operational procedures, looked at the measures these highly skilled professionals used to prevent similar failures in the future.

You'll recall that their research identified two classes of failures: *errors* (defined as the execution of a task either unnecessary or incorrectly carried out), and *problems* (defined as a disruption in the workers' ability to execute a prescribed task because either what was needed was unavailable or something got in the way).

Since 86 percent of the failures were *problems* rather than *errors*, let's focus only on these. Tucker and Edmondson observed that nurses experience five broad categories of problems in performing their work:

- missing or incorrect information,
- missing or broken equipment,
- waiting for a resource (human, supplies or equipment),
- missing or incorrect supplies, and/or
- multiple and simultaneous demands on their time.

Our work with Adaptive Design confirms that these are huge issues for both healthcare providers and management.

Looking through the lens of Rule 1 (Activities), what might one nurse do in an hour's time? Thousands of hours of observation of nurses in real-time reveal that they spend about 43 percent of their time hunting, fetching, clarifying and waiting; 24 percent in administrative activities (e.g., charting and computer data entry); and only 33 percent of their time in direct patient care.

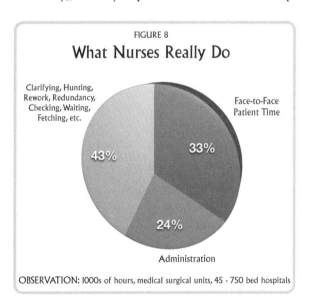

FIGURE 8
What Nurses Really Do

Clarifying, Hunting, Rework, Redundancy, Checking, Waiting, Fetching, etc.

Face-to-Face Patient Time

43%

33%

24%

Administration

OBSERVATION: 1000s of hours, medical surgical units, 45 - 750 bed hospitals

The discovery that nurses spend only one-third of their time in patient care creates a unique, common problem for everyone in healthcare:

- What does the nurse want to do? Take care of patients.
- What does management want the nurse to do? Take care of patients.
- What does the patient want the nurse to do? Take care of patients.

Somehow, problems keep nurses from taking care of patients! A high percentage of the snags were caused by a breakdown in information or material transfer to the nurse. This means connections (Rule 2) and pathways (Rule 3) failed. In the Adaptive Design approach, first, the problems need to be identified quickly. Then they must be concisely described, and solutions developed — all in specified, verifiable and improvable ways. And how should that happen?

Adaptive Design redefines system failures as *problems to be solved*. Find the problem. Then learn, test, validate, fail and improve. That all best comes together when these rules are followed:

Rule 1: All work shall be highly specified as to content, sequence, timing and outcome.

Rule 2: Every customer-supplier connection must be direct, with an unambiguous yes-or-no way to send requests and receive responses.

Rule 3: The pathway for every product and service must be simple and direct.

Each rule requires that activities, connection, and flow paths have built-in tests to signal problems automatically.

The knowledge that underlies the Toyota Production System (and these rules) is built into Adaptive Design for healthcare. While the idea of rules may seem rigid, the common language, structure and discipline actually *create* flexibility that allows the work to adapt to changing circumstances.

This flexibility and adaptability is produced by the last of the four rules, which specifies how to improve.

Rule 4: Any improvement must be made in accordance with the Scientific Method, under the guidance of a teacher, as close to the problem as possible.

How do structure and discipline create flexibility and responsiveness? Chapter 7 will show the *effectiveness* and *power* of Rule 4.

CHAPTER 7

RULE 4: CREATING *IDEAL* HEALTHCARE

"The innovation point is the pivotal moment when talented and motivated people seek the opportunity to act on their ideas and dreams."

– W. ARTHUR PORTER

Why would any adult (let alone an organization) not learn from failure? Tucker and Edmondson's article, entitled "Why Hospitals Don't Learn from Failures," raised more than a few eyebrows.

One significant finding in their study of nursing failures shows why Adaptive Design is such a powerful and necessary tool in the healthcare setting. Tucker and Edmondson cited the extent to which the nurses in the study engaged in what is called "first-order problem solving" — i.e., the worker compensates for a problem by getting the necessary missing or unavailable supplies or information. In first-order problem solving, workers get what they need to complete their work, while never addressing the underlying "root" cause of the problem. Therefore, the chances of a similar problem recurring are never reduced.

Adaptive Design drives improvement to get patients exactly what they need at continually lower cost. Rule 4 fuels the engine that becomes the way to fix healthcare. That's why Rule 4, as modified for healthcare, focuses on improvement through problem solving: **"Any improvement must be made in accordance with the Scientific Method, under the guidance of a teacher, as close to the patient as possible."**[9]

In Adaptive Design, all improvements are driven by the occurrence of a system failure or the opportunity to challenge the status quo to improve. "If it ain't broke, don't fix it!" But if it is broken or can be improved, improve it as quickly and as easily as possible. Improvements should be made *as close as possible* in time and place to the actual work or the source of the problem. Problem solving in Adaptive Design is, therefore, not a meeting room activity. It's part of everyone's daily work on the frontline.

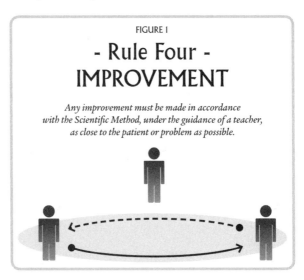

FIGURE 1
- Rule Four -
IMPROVEMENT

Any improvement must be made in accordance with the Scientific Method, under the guidance of a teacher, as close to the patient or problem as possible.

Tucker's and Edmondson's research documented much problem solving. As a matter of fact, problems were so prevalent that nurses could not do their jobs *without* problem solving. They wrote:

> In our research, we found that nurses implemented a short-term fix [what the authors describe as "first-order problem solving"] for the overwhelming majority of failures observed, enabling them to continue caring for their patients without taking any action to try to

---

9 Spear and Bowen state Rule 4 as "...under the guidance of a teacher, at the lowest possible level of the organization." Given the importance of the patient to Adaptive Design, some of our clients have objected to the term "lowest part of the organization." Hence, this change and, in practice, it works, even in non-patient care areas, like finance.

prevent recurrence of similar failures — that is, without promoting organizational learning.

The authors then explained how first-order problem solving often creates new problems elsewhere:

> [F]irst-order problem solving can be counterproductive. It keeps communication of problems isolated so that they do not surface as learning opportunities. Workers rarely inform the person responsible for the problem, which prevents those people from learning that their processes could be improved.

Sometimes, first-order problem solving creates new problems elsewhere. For example, a nurse who can't find a wheelchair to discharge a patient from her unit hunts down an unused wheelchair on another floor. This "first-order fix" does *nothing* to prevent this problem from repeating itself. And, meanwhile, another unit is missing a wheelchair!

In second-order problem solving, the worker and management also take remedial action to address the obstacle. But it doesn't stop there. They also systematically address the root cause of the difficulty, resulting in work-process improvement and institutional learning.

As described in Chapter 5, Clay Christensen's research showed that a successful firm's capability could also be its disability. As such, in healthcare "what is good about us is bad about us." Tucker and Edmondson identified that the very qualities that currently help ensure excellence in patient care (e.g., individual vigilance, concerns regarding unit efficiency and individual empowerment) can leave healthcare workers and management "under-supported and overwhelmed in a system bound to have breakdowns because of the need to provide individualized treatments to patients."

Such consequences inhibit institutional learning and work-process improvement, denying caregivers the ability to address underlying processes in need of revision. Knowledge management in Adaptive Design solves this dilemma by *linking institutional learning to work process improvement.*

How then does a healthcare organization uncover the opportunities presented by system failure? Adaptive Design creates the capability to second-order problem-solve by making it a specified activity embedded into and part of everyone's daily work.

Staying true to our principles, Adaptive Design follows the rules and makes the problem solving activity highly specified as to content, sequence, timing and outcome. In other words, simple, testable and improvable!

Adaptive Design uses Rule 4 to focus improvement on second-order problem solving, beginning with the premise that healthcare systems exist to provide caregivers exactly what they need — when and where they need it. That is the only way Ideal Patient Care can happen. Therefore, not having what a caregiver needs is a problem to be solved.

Steps for second-order problem solving under Adaptive Design are these:

1. The caregiver must immediately identify a problem, i.e., what he or she does not have to meet patient needs Ideally. "If you don't know you have a problem, you can't solve it." (If Yogi Berra didn't say this, he should have!)

2. The caregiver signals that problem to a specified person — the Rule 4 teacher, called the Learner/Leader/Teacher (LLT). Note: I borrowed this title from Toyota because it names a position and evocatively describes what becomes, in Adaptive Design, an important role of management. (Much more about the LLT in later chapters.)

3. The LLT assists the caregiver in getting the patient what is needed, i.e., first-order problem solving.

4. The LLT then facilitates second-order problem solving as "an improvement to be made in accordance with the Scientific Method" (see Appendix One — The Scientific Method).

5. The problem solving is done as close in time and place to the problem as possible. In healthcare, that's as close to the patient (or value creating work in non-patient care areas) as possible. It is only there that the knowledge and creativity of the people directly involved with the problem can be easily accessed.

6. The problem solving is completed as a small, disciplined, structured experiment designed, tested and validated in the course of daily work (see Appendix Two — The A3: Creating Discipline and Structure for Scientific Problem Solving in Healthcare).

The next chapter provides more problem solving details. For now, the main point is this:

By creating rules around activities, connections and pathways, and then specifying the method for making improvements, Adaptive Design tests the validity of each process in the organization every time that process is done.

Both Toyota and healthcare use many powerful process-improvement tools and practices that can be a great platform on which to build adaptive expertise. But Toyota and Adaptive Design are more about developing people than improving processes.

In fact, Toyota and Adaptive Design share a common managerial conviction that **no organization can design perfect processes in complex, dynamic, unpredictable work.** That being true, the solution is to thoughtfully change and adapt any and every process when it inevitably fails.

Empowering that capability requires developing the knowledge, creativity and problem solving ability of every employee in the organization. Making improvements then becomes an everyday occurrence, while the very act of problem solving increases knowledge and learning. This is the knowledge management model of Adaptive Design in healthcare.

An example of how the rules facilitate Adaptive Design as part of daily work can be seen in the following table, taken from one of our clients, a hospital in a large Western health system. Managers and staff carried a plastic version of this card at all times. Any problem in an Activity, Connection or Pathway can be immediately diagnosed by answering the questions on the card.

For example, when assessing a Rule 1 Activity, ask, "Has the content been specified?" If "No," then a problem exists that must be solved quickly and simply.

ACTIVITY	CONNECTION	PATHWAY	HOW TO IMPROVE
(How people work; highly specified)	(How people connect; simple and direct)	(How care is delivered; flows along a simple, specified path)	(People need to know how to change and who is responsible for making changes)
Content?	Who?	Path specified, stable, simple and direct?	Under the guidance of a teacher?
Sequence?	What?	Every resource on path that's needed?	As close to the problems as possible?
Timing?	When?	No resource on path that's not needed?	Done in accordance with the Scientific Method?
Outcome?	How?	Connections follow Rule 2?	Help specified?

This generic approach to managing improvement applies to any complex work environment, and that definitely includes healthcare.

But, how to start? As Tucker and Edmondson identify, healthcare workers and management are "under-supported and overwhelmed in a system bound to have breakdowns because of the need to provide individualized treatments to patients."

How can such obstacles be reasonably and effectively addressed? The answer is, by designing your organization to adapt. You have to start someplace. First, learn to solve small problems when they happen. Then watch how solving the small problems close to the work makes the big problems disappear!

Our Adaptive Design training starts by addressing relatively simple problems. Then we develop and refine the skills of observation and experimentation, continually seeking opportunities for improvement. This type of progressive learning and steady achievement is the hallmark of all human endeavors — from hitting a ball to mastering a musical instrument to managing complex patient care.

Such a personalized learning cycle began, in fact, the day you were born.

Chapters 6 and 7 have provided frameworks, common terms, and language for embedding improvement and innovation into the actions of every person in your organization. I encourage you to return to these chapters frequently as you learn-by-doing.

Now we need to fill in this framework with more specifics about how to create and grow this new culture of performance and innovation. Chapter 8 describes how to start to get patients exactly what they need at continually lower cost with Adaptive Design. In doing so, you will be creating a new order in healthcare.

And if you're wondering what "creating a new order in healthcare" might look like under Adaptive Design, simply reread Bill's story in Chapter 3!

Appendix One —
The Scientific Method: An Overview in Brief

The Scientific Method, central to the principles and practices of Adaptive Design, is how improvements are designed and tested. The Scientific Method has four basic steps described below. This description includes Adaptive Design terms that are defined in the Glossary and will be explicated thoroughly in subsequent chapters:

1. *Observation and description of a phenomenon or a group of phenomena.* In Adaptive Design, the phenomena is healthcare work in progress. Information gathered in this first step is often classified in an effort to simplify and organize what has been found. For example, in medicine, cancer-staging systems are a classification method. In Adaptive Design, dividing the work into Activities, Connections and Pathways acts as the classification system to simplify and organize the complex, dynamic work of healthcare.

2. *Formulation of a theory to explain the observed phenomena.* In Adaptive Design, direct observation and the analysis of the problem to its root cause provides insights into why our current way of working has led to the problem identified. At this stage, a theory is developed that serves as a contingent explanation (the Current Condition) of why things seem to turn out as they do.

3. *This theory (built upon the classification scheme) is then used to predict (hypothesize) what will happen if we worked differently.* In Adaptive Design, the Target Condition is the hypothesized condition, the goal we are trying to reach. In theory, if we achieve the Target Condition, the problem we have identified will not occur.

4. *Performance of experimental tests of the hypothesis.* In physics or the life sciences, several independent researchers may conduct these experimental tests. In Adaptive Design, we test Countermeasures to move from the Current Condition (the way one works now) to the Target Condition (the new way to work). Each Countermeasure is a small experiment testing the ability to change. When the Target Condition has been achieved, a final test is applied by asking, "Yes/No: Is the problem solved?" If the answer is "Yes," we are done. If "No," then we learn more by repeating the process and attempting new solutions.

The Scientific Method rests on the idea that testing the theory may produce unexpected results that do not conform to the original idea of how things should work.

David Lawrence Sundahl and Clayton M. Christensen explain in their Harvard Business School Working Paper "The Process of Building Theory" that, upon identification of an anomaly, it is necessary to cycle back to the earlier classification stage to:

- more accurately describe what the phenomena are and are not,
- revise the classification scheme or devise better classification criteria, and/or
- redefine "what causes what, and why, and under what circumstances."

Christensen and Sundahl report, that "[t]his cycle repeats itself as theory-building researchers, like runners in a relay race, cycle around the track — sometimes keeping the baton as individuals, and sometimes handing the baton to others..."

It is exactly this cycle of continuous improvement through experimental problem solving that lends such power to Adaptive Design. In his article, "No Satisfaction at Toyota" (December 2006, *Fast Company*), Charles Fishman explains that "by constantly questioning how you do things, by constantly tweaking, [Toyota creates] perpetual competitive advantage." As a result of continual experimentation with work processes, "Toyota line employees change the way they work *dozens of times a year.*" (The italics are mine.)

Indeed, science advances by continuously finding holes in its own arguments, rethinking its classification schemes and theories and formulating new or improved views of how things work.

This methodology drives Adaptive Design — and the power of Adaptive Design is that management makes scientific problem solving clear and easy.

Appendix Two —
The A3: Creating Discipline and Structure for Scientific Problem Solving in Healthcare

Toyota developed and refined a simple format to make these experiments and tests reproducible — a form called an A3, based on the size of the paper used to document the experiment (11 x 17 inches). I introduced the A3 to healthcare in 1999. (I have a copy of the first A3 in my files.)

Since then hundreds of people have used this simple form to frame thousands of experiments.

```
┌─────────────────────────────────────────────────────┐
│                                                     │
│  BACKGROUND              TARGET CONDITION           │
│                                                     │
│  CURRENT CONDITION                                  │
│                                                     │
│                                                     │
│                                                     │
│                          COUNTERMEASURES            │
│                                                     │
│  ROOT CAUSE                                         │
│                                                     │
│                                                     │
│                                                     │
│                          TEST                       │
│                                                     │
└─────────────────────────────────────────────────────┘
```

There is nothing magic about an A3. It is just a well-tested tool that simplifies doing structured experiments using the Scientific Method. You will learn more about the Scientific Method and how to use the A3 in healthcare when we do an experiment together in the next chapter.

CHAPTER 8

HARNESSING THE POWER OF CONTINUOUS INNOVATION

"Exact medicine can no more be achieved than exact history, because no human story with a foreordained plot can be anything but a fiction."

– Joseph Schumpeter

The Austrian and Harvard economist Joseph Schumpeter presaged Clayton Christensen's disruptive innovation with his work analyzing the economics of capitalism in the early 20th Century. Schumpeter was blunt in describing what he saw as the huge innovative advantage of capitalism. He named it "Creative Destruction."

In his biography *Prophet of Innovation: Joseph Schumpeter and Creative Destruction* (2007), Thomas K. McCraw, Straus Professor of Business History Emeritus at the Harvard Business School and winner of the Pulitzer Prize for history, gives numerous examples of long-established companies that were wrecked by the irrepressible power of upstart innovators.

The French company Michelin began mass production of the radial tire in the 1940s, setting in motion a sequence of creative destruction that by the 1980s had shattered America's long dominance of the industry. The shift to radials killed-off all the big five tire companies except Goodyear and ended the reign of Akron, Ohio, as the Rubber Capital of the World. An industry-wide culture of complacency, deriving from long success, simply prevented American firms from responding effectively. Sound familiar?

McCraw goes on to cite other notable examples: "During the twentieth century, innovative companies also transformed the 'mature' textile industry by developing rayon, nylon, polyesters, spandex and other synthetic fibers. In steel, the advent of basic oxygen furnaces and mini-mills ended the supremacy of United States Steel, British Steel, and other giant firms." However, he says that "[o]ne of the best examples of all has been the revolutionary Toyota Production System."

In 1960 Toyota Motor Corporation produced only 42,000 cars. By 1980, production had soared to 2.3 million, an increase of 5,240 percent. McCraw points out that Toyota's new production system "not only transformed the making of cars — ending the seven decades of supremacy by Detroit — but also changed the face of manufacturing in general."

Much has been written about Toyota's quality-control systems and its process improvement skills and tools, but (as shown in the last few chapters) the company's real secret is leadership's ability to create an environment where every employee is a powerful unit of creativity and innovation. In this scenario, every manager is a learner, leader and teacher. And, by the way, every employee is a learner and problem solver.

How could a healthcare organization duplicate this success? In my experience, it's simple, but not easy.

Successful organizations often face significant barriers to change and innovation. Yet, Toyota does it continuously and, in contradistinction to the creative destruction Schumpeter identified as essential for innovation, they do it without destroying and rebuilding.

Toyota solves problems in order to improve and innovate. Rather than break old habits, they build new habits. *They change people's minds.* From an organizational perspective, Buckminster Fuller put it well: "You never change things by fighting the existing reality. To change something, build a new model that makes the existing model obsolete."

Make "the existing model obsolete." How?

Experience suggests that the general course of organizational change demands fighting and winning. But Toyota and Adaptive Design don't work that way — and your healthcare organization doesn't have to work that way either. Consider the possibilities in your own setting when you start to *think, act and lead adaptively.*

First and foremost, lead with people! Adaptive Design leaders, like Toyota leaders, *have respect for people!* Specifically, they become increasingly skillful at cultivating humans' natural propensity to adapt, change and improve. These skills have been fundamental to human survival since our earliest emergence as a species, and Adaptive Design's knowledge management methods further develop and leverage that truth on a daily basis.

By nature, humans are problem solvers. Consider the example of a simple home improvement project, e.g., wallpapering a small downstairs bathroom. Maybe you'll begin by consulting a "how-to" book or by discussing the job with someone at the local hardware store that sold you the materials.

As you proceed, not everything you have read or heard helps with the real-life problem of trying to hang wallpaper in a confined space. Maybe you make a few mistakes and have to redo the initial sections, but eventually you begin to *adapt* your methods to the task at hand. Subtly (or perhaps not so subtly), you alter your methods and techniques to improve the quality and efficiency of your work. Maybe a friend or spouse joins in, offering suggestions that further improve the approach. By the end of the project, your natural adaptive ability has taught you more about hanging wallpaper than you knew at the outset.

Often, employees express that their creativity is consistently thwarted by the established organizations in which they work. In comparison, Adaptive Design harnesses and channels this natural, problem solving ability into high-performance, patient-focused innovation.

Clayton Christensen's theories, expressed as disruptive innovation, show clearly that the more successful the company, the more difficult for the organization to transform itself — even if its inability to transform will lead to its destruction.

By studying adaptive innovators, I have distilled five common principles that have the power to meet the innovation needs of large, complex healthcare organizations. The five essential principles are these:

1. Establish an operational framework that fosters trust, optimism, high performance and innovation focused on the patient.
2. Set direction toward a high-reach goal; then eliminate the ambiguities,

assumptions, workarounds and tradeoffs that get in the way.
3. Develop each person's skills, knowledge, creativity and problem solving ability by experimenting and problem solving as frequently as possible.
4. Enhance team focus and performance.
5. Make inquiry and core business execution each person's daily work.

Adaptive Design is a principle-based method. When you put these principles in place and begin to build on them, you automatically start getting patients exactly what they need at continually lower cost. And that means you will be starting to fix healthcare.

The Five Principles in Detail

Each essential principle serves as a guidepost, pointing toward a new way to organize work and generate new and highly transformative levels of innovation. But the principles are only half the story.

You cannot just *think* your way into a new way of acting. You must also *act* your way into a new way of thinking.

As such, coupled with each principle are tools specifically developed for the healthcare setting. These tools will enable management, staff and physicians to put these concepts to work for patients. It is fundamental to the practices of Adaptive Design that principles link to tools that must be integral to, and embedded in, value-adding work. Note the connections in the following examples, as we begin with the general principles:

Principle 1: Establish an operational framework that fosters trust, optimism, high performance and innovation focused on the patient.

High performance and innovation are not two separate things. Innovation that is born out of the work generates high performance. To be highly productive in a changing environment is to be innovative, continuously.

Success breeds success, while good results create trust and optimism. Trust and optimism build resiliency, making it easier to challenge and innovate. Innovation that improves performance closes the loop and builds more trust and optimism. This "virtuous circle" of performance improvement gets better and easier the more it is repeated.

In Adaptive Design, innovation is not a project, not a new strategic plan, and not a new technology. Rather it is the application of insights developed close in time and place to the actual work. And the best part is that, under the guidance of management, it comes from those doing the work!

One problem we consistently see in both large and small healthcare institutions results from the propensity of senior managers to initiate multiple, broad-ranging, resource-intensive programs banked-on to produce big improvements in one or more of four areas: productivity, quality, safety or cost control. A typical result is what I call the "Recurrent Major Initiative Syndrome."

The Recurrent Major Initiative Syndrome has multiple pathologic consequences, the most devastating being Managerial Attention Deficit Disorder (MADD). Managerial focus and leadership are essential in Adaptive Design and that is particularly difficult to achieve with everybody in MADD. If you are a healthcare manager, have you ever found yourself stricken with MADD-ness?

Multiple, complex projects have another effect beyond MADD that can be particularly self-defeating. A big push to increase productivity commonly creates safety issues. In addition, a focus on improving quality can often increase costs. And it's not uncommon for cost control to decrease efficiency or safety.

You may hit your big projects' targets and goals, but does the overall organization improve? Is everyone — staff, physicians, management and patients — better off?

In my experience, big projects fail to make a difference because transformative innovation needs to begin at the most granular level within an organization: Think of the speck of sand that begets a pearl. In Adaptive Design, beginning at a granular level means you may start with a big change — in one small place. Particularly if the organization is large, the first big change begins in one small area.

The Learning Line is the tool we developed to establish this new operational framework of trust, optimism, high performance and innovation. The St. TAH Management Team (Chapter 3) began Adaptive Design by selecting outpatient surgery as the initial Learning Line.

The Learning Line is both a laboratory and an incubator — a single unit that becomes the learning source to safely apply the skills and tools that enable staff to identify, isolate and solve problems. Eventually, the management, staff and physicians will design and test solutions based on their own insights and creativity. The overarching goal is to facilitate real-time problem solving done in the routine course of work.

One might call it powerful *medicine* — on several levels!

Real-time problem solving is an antidote to both big and small problems. Within a complex healthcare delivery system, typically only big problems receive the attention of a busy management team. But large issues are usually only disorientating symptoms of aggregations of multiple small problems.

On the frontline, problems are disaggregated; therefore, they become clearer and more specific. However, without the ability to second-order problem-solve, staff resort to first-order problem solving. First-order problem solving feels good, but it's no cure and only hides the underlying problems. As such, the problems never go away.

Facing variations of the same problem over and over again (e.g., "no consent on the chart") leads to the 4 P's of problem solving: **p**essimism because it's **p**ermanent ("That's just the way it works around here"), **p**ersonal ("If only those people would change"), and **p**ervasive ("It's the same everywhere you go").[10]

Just as ineffective medicine creates pessimistic patients, ineffective problem solving creates pessimistic employees. In such a context, all solutions tend to be difficult, expensive and often illusive! After all, no one can design a perfect process when pessimism reigns. Even if it works, no one believes it.

Leading adaptively means following the Adaptive Design approach of recognizing when systems fail *the moment they fail* and then addressing the problems that caused the failure in *real-time* and in a *disciplined, structured, replicable way*.

Leading adaptively means reciting this mantra, over and over again: **Identify problems quickly, as close in time and place to their occurrence as possible, and then solve them quickly, with a verifiable solution as close to the problem as possible.**

In Adaptive Design, problems simply become opportunities for learning and are considered to be temporary, work-based and local — with *no chance* of becoming permanent, personal and pervasively pessimistic!

Rapid, real-time problem solving creates trust and optimism by contradicting the 4 P's: **P**essimism becomes trust and optimism because everyone discovers problems are not **p**ermanent ("Because we can solve them, they are

---

10 Martin Seligman's research on optimism and pessimism and his book, *Learned Optimism: How to Change Your Mind and Your Life*, have influenced our thinking, work and development of Adaptive Design.

temporary"), and not **p**ersonal ("It's the system, not the people"), and not **p**ervasive ("Problems are local, here and now, because that's the way we solve them").

A Harvard Business School Teaching Case about Toyota's Georgetown, Kentucky, assembly plant tells a revealing story about learning through problem solving. Cars coming off the assembly line were found to have a variety of problems with their seats. At the station where seats were installed, the team installing the back seats were identifying problems and frequently asking for help.

By contrast, workers installing front seats appeared to be encountering no obstacles. The MBA students who discuss this case consistently note real quality and performance issues with the team working on the back seats.

However, the teaching point is this: The Toyota manager's greatest concern was with the team working on the *front* seats. While the back seat team recognized problems and asked for help, the front seat team wasn't finding and solving any problems. And that was a problem!

Culturally, this is the antithesis of what exists in most large organizations, where pointing out problems is almost considered taboo. The Learning Line provides a safe place to embrace problems and develop the awareness that they hold the key to improvement and innovation. In other words, *the Learning Line allows an organization to confront taboos, i.e., deeply held habits, behaviors, processes, and values that block learning and stall innovation.*

Important features of a Learning Line are that it starts,

1. **Small** — It is easier to make a large change in a small place than to make any kind of change in an entire organization.
2. **Simple** — Leaders in healthcare have a penchant to make everything complex. *Don't try to boil the ocean.* I have learned the hard way that the K.I.S.S. principle fits my work perfectly: Keep It Simple, Stupid!
3. **Separate** — as much as possible, from the rest of the organization. Complete separation is rarely possible, but, like the outpatient surgery at St. TAH, by design the Learning Line should be a safe place to test and validate a new way of working that will lead to a new way of thinking about work. The less current thinking and methods impinge on the unit, the better. As Toyota experts say, "Let the work tell you what to do."

Starting is often the hardest part. Creating an operational framework that fosters high performance and innovation through real-time problem solving is not complicated. It's also not easy, simply because it's different. "We don't work this way," is a constant refrain. But the difference makes all the difference! The focus is not process management but *knowledge* management, which is, "learning-by-doing."

Remember: The Learning Line is a location and operational framework that allows workers to *act their way to a new way of thinking.* (More details about Learning Lines are in the subsequent chapters.)

What's the next principle that guides our action? *Know where you are going and remove all roadblocks to getting there.*

Principle 2: Set direction toward a high-reach goal; then eliminate the ambiguities, assumptions, workarounds and tradeoffs that get in the way.

One of the first things essential to starting down the Adaptive Design knowledge management path is to know where you are going. *Ideal Patient Care is the focus.* Your organization starts moving closer to Ideal Patient Care when management sets clear direction.

You might recall that Jane RN at St. TAH stated, "Right at the start, management made it very clear that we were going to move toward Ideal Patient Care — exactly what the patient needs, customized, immediate, safe and with no waste."

Setting direction is an essential attribute of great adaptive leaders. Whenever I talk with individuals who have worked in the start-up of a great innovative company (and certainly among the frontline and management at Toyota), I hear one continual refrain, "We knew where we were going."

Adaptive Design methodology has discovered, tested and validated a powerful approach for setting direction in healthcare: Ideal Patient Care.

First, we establish a Learning Line to solve problems. But how do we know when there is a problem? The management team must set a direction that is meaningful, clear, unambiguous and specific.

The five elements to Ideal Patient Care are easy to state. Just think what you would want for a loved one: First, you don't really want much when you take your child to the doctor. You just want what your son or daughter needs. I think we would all agree, *Ideally,* that means *exactly what's needed, exactly when and where it's needed.* Not more, and certainly not less; just what's needed for your child now.

Next, every person is a unique individual so, Ideally, your child's care would be *customized individually,* specific to his or her needs at that moment.

Also, since healthcare is unpredictable, Ideally, when your child's condition changes, the treatment and activities connected to that care *responds and changes immediately.*

Of course, "Do no harm" has been a standard in healthcare since Hippocrates. As such, you naturally expect your child's care to be *physically and emotionally safe.* In addition, Adaptive Design states that Ideal Care must be safe for all those who deliver it — doctors, nurses, staff, management — everyone must work in an environment that is physically, emotionally and professionally safe.

And, finally, no one wants to see something wasted. So, Ideally, all of your child's care would be delivered *without waste of any resource.* Waste doesn't only refer to material or financial resources, but also to other precious resources, like time, effort, energy, brainpower and people.

In Adaptive Design, management sets strategic direction by making it perfectly clear to everyone that our purpose is to move healthcare toward Ideal Patient Care, meaning care that is,

- exactly what patients need, when and where they need it,
- customized individually,
- immediately responsive to problems or changes,
- safe — physically, emotionally and professionally — for all, and
- provided without wasting any resource.

Any care that is not "Ideal" presents a problem to be solved, an opportunity to learn and a chance to improve the system.

Before examining how Ideal Patient Care guides problem solving, let's first look at four common roadblocks on the adaptive knowledge management path that are far from Ideal: ambiguity, assumptions, workarounds and tradeoffs.

St. TAH's Jane RN said, "We found all sorts of waste, rework and redundancy in what we were doing — and lots of ambiguity, assumptions, workarounds and tradeoffs that got in our way, every day."

Let's look at each one of these obstacles in turn.

Ambiguity is not Ideal!

Ambiguity is inherent in all complex, dynamic and unpredictable work. How many of the written policies, procedures and protocols in your institution are open to multiple interpretations? As a test, try this exercise in your organization:

First, choose some "standard process" (e.g., admission, discharge, medication administration, patient transfer).

Next, put a knowledgeable group of managers and staff together in a room, along with your Policy and Procedures Manual, and ask them to describe and chart the process. Then, observe the actual process with a patient in real-time.

In our experience, the group usually espouses a process that rarely matches the published policies. Furthermore, it never fails to vary from the actual work as observed — and often dramatically. An ambiguous process is no process at all!

Ambiguity is distinct from *vagueness*, which arises when the boundaries of meaning are indistinct. Ambiguity refers to an unclear choice between standard definitions. Would you be surprised to learn that the procedure for administering medications to patients is apt to be highly ambiguous in most organizations?

For example, when a newly graduated nurse joins the team on a medical-surgical unit, she is commonly teamed up with an experienced senior nurse to teach her the procedures for administering medications. Generally, the senior nurse runs her through the process several times, showing her how to operate the automated drug dispensing machine, how to complete the forms necessary to document the process and how to prepare the medications for dispensing.

After working awhile under the tutelage of the senior nurse, the new nurse has the procedure down cold. She is ready to work independently. What do you suppose is the likelihood that, if the new nurse had been trained by a different senior staff member, she would have been shown the exact same procedure? The probability is low.

There may be as many ways to administer medication as nurses on the floor. Moreover, what is the likelihood that the new nurse will replicate the process exactly as demonstrated? Too often, the communication regarding our critical work processes in healthcare resembles the children's "telephone" game where a group of kids sit in a circle and whisper a phrase or sentence into the ear of the adjacent child. With each repetition, the message becomes more distorted.

The traditional approach to solving this process variation is to attempt to eliminate ambiguity by standardizing the work — usually by pulling together experts who can survey and codify industry-standard best practices. Another option is to buy technology that forces workers to follow a specific pathway and method.

That's the conventional wisdom; Toyota and Adaptive Design take an unconventional approach. Rather than eliminate ambiguity by designing perfect processes, we identify when ambiguity causes a problem and then eliminate that ambiguity as part of the solution.

For example, consider how Toyota deals with a requisitioned part that fails to arrive on time. The person who needs the part will signal a problem to his dedicated resource for problem solving. They then think Rule 2: *Every customer-supplier connection must be direct*, with simple ways to identify if the connection is defect-free. Immediate assessment shows that the request for the part was specific as to *what* was needed, by *whom* and *where*, but it failed to identify *when* the part was needed. The ambiguity therefore becomes immediately apparent and is quickly resolved by redesigning the requisition to include the "when."

At Toyota, an employee with an ambiguity problem immediately signals a specified person, i.e., for the front line, their team leader (Learner/Leader/Teacher). Then the necessary resources are put to work finding a short and long-term solution during the course of regular work. Toyota is famous for "stopping the line." But what most don't realize is that, in one study, **workers solved 12 problems for every one problem that stopped the line**. "Stopping the line" is only the tip of the iceberg of problem solving in the course of work.

Notice this comparable healthcare example: A physician writes an order with unclear timing for a preoperative antibiotic. For years, I have watched nurses and pharmacists bend-over backwards to clarify this ambiguity by trying to decipher handwriting, guess at intentions, look up options in a drug reference, ask someone what the doctor usually does, and so on.

Such a problem is identical to that of the delayed part delivery on the Toyota assembly line, but the expectation of "no ambiguity" has not been clearly established in healthcare. Nor has the capability to solve the problem been developed. The response to unclear timing for a medication on a Learning Line might be to notify the physician immediately. The physician then becomes aware of the problem and the patient gets what is needed. But that's also a first-order solution.

The missed timing could happen again tomorrow with another physician. A second-order solution might then be to work with the Learning Line physicians to redesign the preoperative orders, so that the timing of antibiotics becomes unambiguously part of a physician's work in writing the order.

The first problem I encountered in testing Toyota's adaptive knowledge management principles in healthcare, back in 1999, was — no surprise — a missing medication. Examining the root cause, I discovered that the physician had written an incomplete, ambiguous order. (This will also be no surprise to any of my nurse or pharmacist readers.)

Developing the root cause, I discovered no general agreement on what constituted a complete medication order. Pharmacists, nurses, physicians and managers all had different ideas and disagreed even among themselves. Now that's ambiguity!

Under Adaptive Design, such an ambiguity becomes immediately evident as a problem and is resolved by a solution created during work, specifically designed in the context of what this patient needs — *now*!

I will detail the actual problem solving steps in the next chapter, but suffice it to say that if this case occurred at St. TAH, Jane RN would signal the problem immediately to the specified person charged with problem solving. (Remember what happened when Bill received the wrong discharge medication?) A disciplined, structured approach challenges staff and physicians to devise a solution that makes it easy for the physician to do the right thing, e.g., write a complete order for pre-op antibiotics that includes timing.

As I will detail in the next chapter, a simple, disciplined, structured method creates a prototype solution that would be tested in the workplace and improved until a stable solution is found. All this happens on a Learning Line in the course of work. Meetings are rare and called only to solve a specific problem. The solution's validation comes by demonstrating that this antibiotic timing problem has been solved because an ambiguous order does not recur.

The organization "learns" by identifying a system failure and immediately rectifying it in a structured, replicable way. If the problem does recur, that's just another problem to solve.

This, obviously, is not "Standard Operating Procedures" in healthcare. Under Adaptive Design the Learning Line becomes the place to learn how to do something different; the alternative is more of the same.

During one recent observation of medication administration, the drawer of the automated drug dispensing machine tore open the blister package of a Schedule V drug, requiring the nurse to reseal the damaged packaging with cellophane tape before returning it to the drawer. Being a dedicated professional, she solved the problem on the spot. In other words, she engaged in first-order problem solving and then went on with her work.

We all encourage this kind of immediate response to problems in healthcare. However, no learning occurs. As the Tucker and Edmondson article documented, unfortunately the same problem will arise again — and again.

Adaptive Design establishes the expectation that, because ambiguity must be eliminated, the capability to identify and do so is created as **part of the everyday work** — without meetings, policies or taskforces!

When ambiguity causes a problem, signal it, find the root cause and engineer a verifiable solution. Simultaneously, the ambiguity is resolved.

Assumptions are not Ideal!

Everyone makes assumptions. In the 17th Century, John Locke, the father of English empiricism, observed that if we find the grass wet in the morning, we can assume it rained during the night. But maybe the cause was morning dew or, in today's world, your underground sprinkler system.

Many management decisions are also based on assumptions. Managers assemble the best data available, conduct a rigorous analysis, form a conclusion and make a decision. But how well informed are these decisions in the complex, dynamic and unpredictable environment of modern healthcare?

I recently observed a hospital task force charged with the job of deciding how many managers the organization should have. They bought "Best Practice" information from various consulting organizations and discovered data that told them to create a patient to management ratio of 6.2:1.

Now, since everybody knew the "benchmark," everyone felt comfortable establishing this ratio. The benchmarking consultants were assumed to be credible; the results were assumed to be current (actually they were more than one year old) and representative of this hospital's market, range of services, patient population, and on and on — one assumption after another. But, it's a benchmark — it has to be right!

My assumption? The data was most likely useless. There was absolutely no evidence that the benchmark was relevant to this hospital's current situation.

What do you think? I know what Toyota thinks. Their unique approach eliminates assumptions. They simply say: If you saw it happen, you know it happened. Anything else is an assumption.

I can remember many times in my TPS training that, when reporting an incident, I was inevitably asked, "How do you know that happened?" If my answer was, "I was told so," or "This is the way the system works," I was always sent back with the admonition to (as Toyota experts say over and over again) "Go, look, and see."

Assumptions are eliminated by not focusing on the work "as espoused," but on the work as observed. In Adaptive Design we don't create solutions based on aggregated data and workers' reports. Problems are solved in real-time, in the workplace, using information based upon direct observation.

How might such an approach eliminate assumptions in healthcare? Let's examine a "simple" problem – at least, presumably simple.

One hospital engineered a well thought-out procedure for medication orders to be faxed from the nursing station to the pharmacy downstairs. It was embraced as a great time-saver and provided important documentation of medication requests. But in the course of starting a Learning Line in the unit, it was discovered that medications were occasionally not available when needed, in spite of a "fax-received" confirmation.

After the fax was sent and the confirmation automatically generated, the assumption was that the pharmacy had received exactly what it needed. It was also assumed that the fax generated the appropriate response from the pharmacy. In an assessment of problems, we discovered that faxes were occasionally misdirected, lost or stalled. Sometimes a fax even generated a different response from the pharmacy than what was desired.

Therefore, "I faxed the order. The confirmation has been received. The patient will get the med" might not be a fact. This exact scenario has been observed in computer-generated orders. The presumption that the sophistication and expense of advanced technology will solve the "med administration problem" is widespread, but in my experience not necessarily true. It is only an assumption; and, unfortunately, a very expensive one.

The following are some examples involving a nursing staff, the hospital pharmacy and some enlightening problems:

1. One day a nurse, despite having faxed an order for a single dose, one-time medication, was unable to get it from the Pyxis machine (one of several brands of automated, computer-controlled medication dispensing devices) when needed for a patient. This was on a Learning Line and her manager's work had been redesigned to support problem solving, so the nurse signaled the problem and faxed a second order. The manager observed the actual process in the pharmacy and discovered the computer automatically deleted a one-time medication order if a nurse did not "pick" the medication within

four hours. This was a hidden glitch in the computer system because only pharmacists had access to the screen that showed the order, and they had no way of knowing the medication order automatically timed-out. The pharmacy was able to adjust the system to allow access to one-time medications for a more appropriate time period.

2. Another nurse could not get an ordered medication from the Pyxis and signaled a problem. This time, when investigated, the manager discovered the fax was only assumed to have been sent. The pharmacy fax line was 7899 and, as she reviewed the fax log, she noticed there was a fax failure to 7789. The "fax incomplete" report came two minutes later when the busy nurse or unit clerk had moved on to a new task. The manager had *assumed* everyone knew how to use the auto-dial on the machine. She eliminated this assumption by creating a step-by-step "how to fax to the pharmacy" guide and taping it right on the fax machine.

3. Days later a nurse signaled she could not get a one-time medication for a patient from the Pyxis. Confidently, the manager *assumed* she knew the solution and went to the pharmacy to find out what was wrong with the computer. She and the pharmacy staff discovered that it was not a computer problem, but rather the pharmacy staff did not know that particular order was for them. The order sheets contain pharmacy and non-pharmacy orders. Unit clerks should put a checkmark in a designated column for all pharmacy orders, but in this case the fill-in unit clerk had left the box unchecked. The work was redesigned so that temporary unit clerks would understand their work *without assumptions*.

The only way to rid your organization of false and misleading assumptions is to get the facts by direct observation of the work in progress and responding immediately to problems when the work cannot be completed as expected.

Not one of these problems would have been solved if it had not been investigated immediately, because there was no way the needed information could have been discovered later. Information, like a vegetable, *spoils* over time.

But it's not just information! Relationships and morale also suffer. At St. TAH, prior to Adaptive Design, Jane RN described how the nurses assumed the doctors were the problem, and the doctors assumed the nurses were to blame. Both groups blamed management — and everybody thought overly-demanding patients were the problem!

Toyota teaches, the story of St. TAH's Adaptive Design illustrates and our experience confirms, that the only way to rid your organization of false and misleading assumptions is by direct observation of the work in progress and by making immediate responses to problems when the work cannot be completed as expected.

There is no substitute for direct observation.

Workarounds are not Ideal!

Workarounds are endemic in healthcare. As a vascular surgeon, I did or caused workarounds almost daily. As a matter of fact, hospitals tend to highly praise staff and physicians who are the best at workarounds.

See if this conversation doesn't sound familiar: "That Mary, she's the greatest nurse. She always locates the chart, gets the consent I forgot, orders the missing CBC, finds the X-ray, corrects the instrument card, remembers my favorite Metzenbaum surgical scissors, locates the anesthesiologist, reminds me I am in Room Two today, rounds up the family, gets me to see the consult, finds me for the next case, *etc., etc.* That Mary, she's the best."

Yet all these workarounds are only hiding the underlying system failures that some day will unexpectedly blossom into a big problem. The scenario has been repeated over and over again: one small problem leads to another, then another. Ultimately, the results will be big system failure, perhaps a "sentinel event," or worse, everyone's great fear of harm to an innocent worker or patient.

Although you would never classify the following as a sentinel event, it's indicative of the thinking that creates one. A nurse, a bit behind in his work, was busy changing bed linens. He stripped the sheets from the bed in Room 302 and went to the linen closet for fresh sheets. There were none. He checked his watch, sighed deeply, then clicked his tongue. He knew he should call housekeeping, but it was just faster to fix it on his own. He walked quickly to an adjacent unit, entered their linen closet and took a pile of sheets and pillowcases, enough for Room 302. Mission accomplished!

Here's the hitch: Not only is this first-order problem solving, but Nurse Jones has caused a downstream problem in the adjacent unit. It will run short of linen sooner than expected and probably well before the scheduled restocking. Where do you suppose someone on that unit will go to find the necessary supplies in a pinch? How will housekeeping ever know how much each unit needs? Finally, it contributes to the 4 P's (personal, permanent and pervasive pessimism) and a culture that accepts mediocrity, as long as it doesn't hurt anyone.

How about the parking problem in Chapter 3? Bill was pleased to learn about all the ways that Jane RN and her colleagues had improved care, but he couldn't have cared less about Core Measures. What really amazed him was his own parking space. How did that capability develop? It was the parking valet's discovery that his whole job was a workaround of the complex, aggregate problem of patient flow. When problem solving began to clarify and eliminate the complexity, his job could be redesigned from workaround valet to problem solving parking coordinator.

And what did Bill see that pleased him so? Just his own parking place.

Workarounds are what is done to get patients what they need ASAP without ever getting to the root cause of the problem. Staff "solve" the linen shortage problem every day — which is exactly the problem! In Adaptive Design, staff, physicians and management *look at workarounds as the hard work people do to get patients what they need without an easy way to second-order problem-solve.*

Tradeoffs are not Ideal!

Often, tradeoffs take the form of workarounds at the management level. In efforts to improve quality, actions are taken or policies are instituted that ultimately increase costs. Cost control measures, more often than not, result in staff reductions and a corresponding decrease in quality or the extent of services offered.

I recall my own experience as a health system executive in the Pacific Northwest. After a major re-engineering initiative came widespread staff cutbacks. I was one of the few senior executives to oppose the move. Nevertheless, all departments were affected and I was forced to let-go (among others) a highly qualified senior manager in the social services department who had refused to go along with the cuts mandated for her department.

A few weeks later, I found myself in the emergency department at 3:00 A.M. trying, without much success, to deal with a social services nightmare — a problem I lacked the resources and skill to solve. That delay obstructed ED flow, led to an unnecessary hospitalization, ruined not just my night but that of the multiple people I called upon for help, and forced me to postpone a long and difficult surgery the following day. And finally, of course, we failed to meet this patient's social service needs Ideally. Was this a sentinel event? Not by usual definitions. However, clearly this was an unrecognized sentinel of a troubled system.

The problem is that healthcare is by nature complex, dynamic and unpredictable. Therefore, best intended efforts have unintended consequences. Too often, when we try to control costs we sacrifice quality, safety or outcomes. In an effort to increase safety, we sometimes can make the work more complicated. We increase quality, but often at a higher cost. These are all tradeoffs.

What Adaptive Design promises is a mechanism to achieve higher quality *and* productivity *and* lower costs, without sacrificing our most valuable asset — people, along with their knowledge and creativity. No tradeoffs!

Jane RN and colleagues at St. TAH broke the upward cost/quality cycle by eliminating the assumption that quality costs more. How did they do it?

Management, instead of expending capital to solve a problem, focused on return on assets (ROA). Their constant challenge was to break the habit of buying more resources and, instead, generate more value from current resources.

For example, at the time Bill had his surgery, Jane RN was testing the innovative concept of the "Personal Nurse." And where did the extra nursing resources come from? Not from hiring more staff, but by capturing the knowledge, creativity and problem solving ability of current staff to redesign their own work to better meet patient needs Ideally.

Take another look at Figure 8 in Chapter 6. I'll be somewhat radical and say that, perhaps, we don't need more nurses at the point-of-care. Rather we need to capture RN knowledge, creativity and problem solving ability to progressively eliminate the administrative work and first-order problem solving that keeps nurses away from patients. Knowledge-management and problem solving in the course of work will deliver what the nurses want, what the managers want, and what the patients want — more *patient-focused nursing time*!

As one hospital executive told me in a large mountain state hospital after he had a chance to observe nursing work in real-time, "Those nurses aren't treating patients, they're treating the system!" I agree. So let's get back to treating patients.

The key point is this: Tradeoffs are nothing more than the little Dutch boy putting his finger in the dike. New problems are certain to resurface elsewhere in the organization.

Adaptive Design eliminates tradeoffs!

The most reliable way to eliminate ambiguity, assumptions, workarounds and tradeoffs in your organization is through the application of the third essential principle.

Principle 3: Develop each person's skills, knowledge, creativity and problem solving ability by experimenting and problem solving as frequently as possible.

In a typical community hospital, 1,000 to 2,000 human brains function within the organization. This represents a tremendous reservoir of skill, knowledge, creativity and problem solving ability. The goal is to develop and use the talent and potential of everyone — all in the pursuit of Ideal Patient Care. You create better problem solvers when people problem-solve often. Humans get very good at what they do frequently. To gain better skills, knowledge, creativity and problem solving, increase the opportunities for problem solving.

You've heard the cliché, "We must empower our people." Unfortunately, it almost never happens. Imagine the benefits if an organization could develop true internal entrepreneurship.

At St. TAH, Jane RN explained how they were able to make so many improvements. Before Adaptive Design, everybody assumed management found the answers and the staff did the work. But soon they learned that the four rules created discipline and structure for problem solving, which needed to be done on the frontline. If it couldn't be done there, then certainly management had to become involved — but only then. The primary tool used to develop this capacity was *rapid, real-time problem solving*, done at the point-of-care. First, the direction needed to be perfectly clear.

Again, Ideal Patient Care is:

- exactly what the patient needs, when and where he/she needs it,
- customized individually,
- immediate response to problems or changes,
- safe — physically, emotionally and professionally — for all, and
- no waste of resources.

Rather than trying to design a perfect system in the abstract, specific steps are taken to problem-solve any system that is not Ideal *as a scientific experiment*. Ideal Patient Care merely provides direction, because less-than-ideal healthcare is not a secret well hid. It's apparent to everyone.

Ideal Patient Care is not a target to hit, nor a goal to be achieved. Rather, it's a guiding principle, a purpose for the work. Like the bright and consistent North Star, Adaptive Design can be used to chart a direction or reorient when employees wander off course.

Peter Senge, in his seminal work *The Fifth Discipline: The Art & Practice of The Learning Organization*, describes this kind of direction-setter as an "attractor goal," something that pulls the organization forward in the proper direction.

Healthcare is ultimately about the patient. As a result, striving for Ideal Patient Care *should take place by problem solving as close to the patient as possible. After all, there is no better place to add value for the patient.*

Ideal Patient Care has been tested in dozens of different healthcare environments over the last eight years, and each time we find one major attribute: "Ideal" is meaningful to everyone in the workplace.

"Core values," as important motivators, are often dependent on the context. Like beauty, they may exist only in the eye of the beholder. For example, what is *excellence* to you? How about *stewardship* or *collegiality* or *collaboration*? The definitions may vary widely by individual. By contrast, Ideal Patient Care can be defined in a much more binary fashion. Either it is Ideal — or it's not!

- Did the patients get exactly what they needed? yes/no
- Was it customized to them individually? yes/no
- Was there an immediate response to problems or changes? yes/no
- Was it physically safe? yes/no
- Was it emotionally safe? yes/no
- Was it professionally safe? yes/no
- Did it involve any waste of resources? yes/no

Rather than trying to send in a team that will design Ideal Patient Care for a healthcare organization (an impossible task, I would say), Adaptive Design empowers the staff, physicians and management. *They* tell *us* when they do not have what they need to meet patient care needs Ideally. When a need is unmet, it's time to signal a problem. The system should meet the needs of patient care *Ideally*. The patients and staff members themselves are relied upon to indicate problems to solve.

Our previous examples show how this works. Take Mary, our wonderful nurse in the previous workaround section. By using the definition of Ideal Patient Care, let's evaluate her work. She always does these things:

- Locates the missing chart. (That missing chart's a problem: How can I provide Ideal Patient Care if there is no chart?)
- Gets the forgotten consent. (That's a problem.)
- Orders the missing CBC. (Another problem.)
- Finds the X-ray. (Another problem.)
- Corrects the instrument card. (Problem!)
- Remembers the favorite Metzenbaum surgical scissors. (Why does she have to remember? Why can't the system just get it there? Because this is a problem!)
- Locates the anesthesiologist. (Are you seeing this as a problem?)
- Reminds me that I am in room two today. (Why don't I know where I need to be? Trust me; this is a big problem for physicians.)
- Rounds up the family. (Why do they need rounding up?)
- Gets me to see the consult. (Why don't I know what to do?)
- Finds me for the next case. (I suspect you get the point.)

That Mary, she is "the best" at workarounds. And, you know, I bet she would be a great second-order problem solver too, if ever she had a chance.

However, in a typical hospital, Mary would not be encouraged to recognize these workarounds as system problems. Instead, she would be encouraged to first-order problem-solve one at a time, in isolation. "That Mary — she's the greatest nurse. She takes care of all the little problems and only lets me know about the big ones."

With Adaptive Design, anything less than Ideal Patient Care is a problem to be addressed at the system level as a small, but structured, scientific experiment. Why? *So it does not happen again.*

The power of such directed, real-time problem solving cannot be overestimated. Managers and staff gain control over problems that previously seemed unsolvable. And the creative and corrective insights are "owned" by the frontline and their managers. This means a total buy-in when this new way of working succeeds and problems are solved.

As Jane RN at St. TAH said, "It is now clear that identifying problems and participating in solutions is everyone's responsibility. We take that responsibility very seriously. But, honestly, now we don't have to think about it. We just do it as part of our work." This system creates accountability.

Moreover, problem solving in real-time with the goal of achieving Ideal Patient Care has the ability to address multiple and very different obstacles simultaneously, such as: quality, safety, finance and process issues. And where it counts most — in the workplace!

Go back to Mary's list of tradeoffs and workarounds. The first one (Locates the patient's chart), I think we would agree is a *quality* problem. And is it a *safety* problem? Well, yes, if we are missing important information. How about *financial*? Absolutely, if it slows throughput or wastes resources. An *organizational* or *process* obstacle? Well, think about it.

Clearly, each tradeoff and workaround in Mary's list actually represents combined quality, safety, financial and organizational issues as well as process obstacles, which could all be simultaneously addressed by Adaptive Design through problem solving in the course of work.

Finally, learning never stops. As Jane RN described, "If you solve the small problems close to you, the big problems tend to go away." The initial, and sometimes small, successes achieved early-on lead to new and more dramatic successes and insights as experience is gained. This creates "cycles of increasing returns" for both workers and the organization.

Recurrent success engenders greater trust and optimism.

The cycle becomes *continuous and self-renewing* as a positive feedback loop for *sustaining improvement.*

Principle 4: Enhance team focus and performance.

In healthcare, no one person can do everything. Therefore, the fourth essential principle reinforces working in ways that enhance team focus and performance. Focus is key, since the nature of the work will change due to the dynamic nature of healthcare. Adaptive Design creates clarity, since the focus is always on *this problem now.*

Teams that assemble to solve a specific problem should, in fact, be ephemeral. In other words, they dissolve after a specific job is done and reorganize into a new configuration, with a personnel and skill-set change appropriate to the new problem that needs to be solved.

The motto for Adaptive Design is to use only the resources needed to solve this one problem now. Once that happens, the team disperses back to its regular work. To keep a team functioning after a completed goal is a waste of resources — and that's not Ideal.

In the following example, notice how a focused interdisciplinary team solved a seemingly intractable problem and captured unrealized revenue in the process.

A large city hospital on the East Coast had an unusual problem because, unlike typical prospective payment or DRGs (hospital Medicare payments based on patient diagnosis), it was reimbursed for specific charges on uncompensated care. As the region's "safety-net provider," the organization saw increasing numbers of patients with no insurance or Medicaid coverage. For the hospital to be appropriately reimbursed, supplies or equipment used for the indigent must be identified.

A Learning Line was established in the operating room's post anesthesia care unit (PACU). The staff was taught to note when they were missing necessary items to meet patient care needs *Ideally*. Adaptive Design experiments empowered their second-order problem solving. In the end, their expectations changed. They *expected* the system to work and responded to problems when it did not. Just like Jane RN and her coworkers at St. TAH, they were becoming "intolerant of mediocrity."

One day, as an RN replaced a Foley catheter (a device commonly used to drain the urinary bladder), she discovered a problem. She knew her hospital depended on reimbursement for supplies for uncompensated care. She also knew that, without this reimbursement, the hospital would have difficulty fulfilling its mission to serve the poor. So not knowing how to charge for the catheter was a problem.

She immediately signaled her problem and, with the help of her LLT, a quick analysis showed that:

1. No one in the PACU could agree on what and how to charge. (**Ambiguity**)
2. Such small costs were not considered significant. (**Assumption**)
3. When they did charge, they guessed how to do it. (**Assumption** and **Workaround**)
4. These low cost items were not worth the time to sort out because of all the other important things to do. (**Assumption** and **Tradeoff**)

The PACU nurses were not alone in their assumptions. The finance department agreed that this was a small dollar item and they had much bigger fish to fry. Who cares about whether to charge for a catheter?

However, Adaptive Design creates new expectations by making it easy to bring the resources together to solve a problem quickly. In that previous case, staff, management and the finance department quickly discovered that the PACU lacked a reliable charge-identification method. In addition, often charges identified were disallowed by the State Medical Assistance Office due to inadequate documentation. The nursing staff not only contributed their expertise, they were appalled to find themselves part of the hospital's revenue shortfall.

The finance team discovered the frontline to be a powerful resource of knowledge and creativity to solve a chronic problem they could never have gotten their arms around on their own. Ultimately, the new charge capture process extended to the rest of the OR. The result? Big items were being missed well beyond Foley catheters, with revenue totaling $625,000, direct to the bottom line — in just the first month!

Following this amazing finding, the "charge capture team" dispersed, and everyone returned to his or her regular jobs. Why? Problem solved! Don't forget that teams are created to help solve specific problems only when extra resources are needed. No problem, no team.

Principle 5: Make inquiry and core business execution each person's work, every day.

St. TAH's information technology department was not the only one responsible for the problems with its information system. This was everyone's problem. That led to the Ideal Health Card, a unique, simple and low-cost technological accelerator that St. TAH did not purchase and roll out, but created itself.

Making it clear to everyone and every team that inquiry and core business execution is job-one every day will supercharge your organization. It tells *every* employee that he or she is important and critical to the success of the business. Plus, it opens the door to developing each person's full potential.

- Every person's job is important.
- Completing every person's job is important.
- Everyone helps brings the organization closer to *Ideal*.

If you cannot complete your work Ideally, that's a problem you are accountable to identify and one that the organization must help you solve.

For example, a new part-time housekeeper is empowered and also expected to ask questions if she can't do what should be done or if she believes her work can be improved. Her job is core to the organization, because *people* make the difference. In adaptive knowledge management, respect for people is the number one priority.

In Adaptive Design, every person is important, and every person's job is important. These are not management clichés: they are authentic, actual and real principles to be reiterated daily.

In Adaptive Design, *we mean what we say and we say what we mean.* And this authenticity is confirmed by our actions. Because this housekeeper knows more than anyone else about her work, that knowledge is key to the organization's success.

Adaptive Design also places a great responsibility on each employee. Not only is a housekeeper expected to identify problems, the Adaptive Design method and her coworkers hold her accountable to do so. The next step is to use that intimate knowledge of the work proactively to question the "why and how" of the job. For example:

- Why do I have to mop this way when another technique gets the floor cleaner, faster?
- How can I find out about patient discharges sooner so I can turn over the room more effectively?
- Why do we throw away these pillows?

The freedom and capability of each person to ask the necessary questions to complete a job Ideally is at the core of Adaptive Design's success.

Adaptive Design summons the entire organization to work toward a common purpose in a unique way and then provides a specific set of rules, skills and tools, along with the know-how to deliver on these principles. Any organization or leader that can create the skills and capabilities needed to deliver on these five principles is going to be successful.

The next chapter will guide you on a tour through a real-life hospital that adopted and learned knowledge management through Adaptive Design. When the principles and practices are applied, the differences in healthcare practice, employee morale and patient care are nothing less than astounding.

CHAPTER 9

"GETTING IT DONE:" REAL-TIME LESSONS FROM ADAPTIVE ORGANIZATIONS

"The ultimate difference between a company and its competition is, in fact, the ability to execute."

– LARRY BOSSIDY

"Toyota is different," Hajime Ohba, the former head of Toyota Supplier Support Center for North America, explained to me. "First, we change people's minds, then develop their natural talents. Everything else flows from that."

Some years ago I had the opportunity to dine with Mr. Ohba. In visiting about Toyota's unique management methods, he basically described it this way: Other consultants ("experts") implement new methods, structures, tools and technology, expecting *these* to change the people. And it works, usually, for a while.

"However," Ohba explained, "the people always go back to the way they were or where the work takes them."

That's why Toyota's (and Adaptive Design's) methods are (as Ohba said so simply and elegantly), "different."

In the healthcare setting, Adaptive Design consultants teach that improvement must first begin by changing people's minds. A tall order, you say? An impossible task? Experience proves it is not necessarily so, especially when change provides the opportunity for personal development integrated into the very fabric of the workplace.

When patient care can be refined and optimized in real-time, both rapidly and demonstrably, the work life of those providing the care changes drastically. Real-time problem solving is the key, starting with these three concepts:

1. **It is almost impossible to design a perfect healthcare process**. Therefore, don't worry about perfection. Just set a starting point and use Adaptive Design to begin to identify failure as a marvelous opportunity to improve.

2. **Like an exercise program, the more you practice Adaptive Design, the greater the return.** Adaptive Design is not a one-time fix — it is work-place fitness.

3. **Healthcare is a wonderful, life-giving profession and business.** Adaptive Design's focus on the patient returns pride, purpose and commitment to the front line and rejuvenates the management team.

Having served in healthcare for 37 years, I well remember when it was a pleasure to care for people. Unfortunately, many confess that it's no longer as fun — and certainly not as rewarding. You can't imagine my pleasure when I see a nurse with a twinkle in her eye who says, "We just solved a problem that has plagued us for years and we did it in a matter of hours." Making that kind of a difference is fun!

SIDEBAR

Thoughts on Reading about Learning-By-Doing

Adaptive Design is a simple concept. The following sums it up:

1. **Focus on just one thing:** Meeting individual patient needs Ideally.
2. **Develop people:** The number one resource.
3. **Understand the work:** Eliminate assumptions, ambiguity, work-arounds and tradeoffs.
4. **Maintain stability:** If it works, don't change it.
5. **Problem-solve to improve:** If it doesn't work or can be improved,

that improvement should happen quickly and simply, designed as an experiment and accomplished as much as possible as part of everyone's daily work.

But disruptive innovation teaches that any concept, regardless of how simple, is not necessarily easy to execute if it differs from current practice. Conventional wisdom is, well, conventional. Although comfortably familiar, it is definitely not thinking "out of the box." Thinking out of the box in an established organization is a lot harder than most people realize.

Once acquired, Adaptive Design is a method and skill-set that makes creative thinking an everyday occurrence. It is not a mystery, but it does require learning-by-doing. For example, the components of Adaptive Design run as common threads through the best of today's leadership and management literature (see the Bibliography). But just reading will not get you there. You must actually *do* to *learn*.

For those of you who are sports-minded, here's a familiar metaphor for learning-by-doing. You want to learn a new sport; say golf, bike riding, fly-fishing, soccer, hang-gliding or lawn darts — pick a sport, any sport. Now, read all the books you can get your hands on and go to several workshops. Would you be even a modestly competent practitioner, let alone an expert? In my experience, the answer is no.

Adaptive Design requires knowledge, but, more importantly, it is a skill. And skills are acquired and developed by doing, discovering and improving. As Toyota says, "You cannot know until you see; you cannot see until you do." Learning-by-doing under the guidance of a teacher is like observation; there is no substitute.

Learning-by-doing is particularly challenging for senior managers working in the traditional top-down, expert-based, process-focused, 20th Century "industrial" management model we are so very accustomed to. As an experienced hospital CEO told us in the early years of our work, "A CEO can't be green." And she was not talking about the environment. Overcoming this deeply engrained value-set and making it safe to acknowledge "senior management should not know how to fix everything," is essential.

It becomes safe when it is emphasized that it is a *waste of valuable managerial and executive time and resources* for senior management to work on big problems that can be disaggregated and solved lower in the organization.

Senior management then learns to lead adaptively by developing and coordinating problem solving that is moved continually closer to the problem as it happens.

Therefore, to execute effectively, senior management needs the opportunity to learn-by-doing also. (I will develop more on the management role and learning in the next chapter.)

Execution

The hard work of moving your organization from where it is now to where you want it to be is called *execution*. Execution means closing the gap between intention, plans and reality, and Adaptive Design is all about execution. And, in my experience, execution is the missing link for most organizations.

Organizations using Adaptive Design make a difference by executing — by getting it done — because Adaptive Design is:

- *A System* — get things done by questioning, problem solving and following-through.
- *A Discipline* — requires a deep understanding of who, what, where, when, why and how.
- *A Method* — structured skills and tools.
- *The Link* — between the core processes, strategy, operations and people.
- *Sustainable Results* — creates a high performance culture (a new DNA).

Organizations start executing with Adaptive Design when they learn-by-doing. The goal is to create adaptive organizational independence — not consultant dependence. Here are some lessons learned by adaptive healthcare organizations that are executing at the point-of-care.

Execution: Starting to learn-by-doing.

As described in Chapter 8, management and staff begin to learn the principles of Adaptive Design by finding a place to establish a Learning Line — an operational framework that fosters trust, optimism, high performance and innovation.

The first step in creating a Learning Line is to bring together a cross-section of people who understand best how things work in the institution. Usually, five or six units within the organization end up being considered good candidates. The team then reaches a consensus about an ideal place for a Learning Line.

In choosing a starting point, the **five most important variables** are these:

1. stable staff and management,
2. some local dissatisfaction with current methods and management open to learning,
3. less work complexity (a unit providing fewer services with fewer people is easier to change because there are fewer moving parts),
4. meaningful as a learning site for the rest of the organization, and
5. the opportunity for improvement (e.g., a big medical-surgical unit will show great gains despite its complexity).

Of these five factors, **stable staff and management are the most important**. Adaptive Design progressively changes minds and develops people. That's more difficult if the employees keep changing. It's also easier to change minds when the current staff and management feel some level of dissatisfaction with their work environment. Dissatisfaction helps open the door for innovation. As in chronic disease management, "readiness to change" is essential to doing things differently.

After deciding on a Learning Line, management identifies one or two people to be their first Learners/Leaders/Teachers (LLTs). These LLTs are the foundation for the organization's learning, since they will lead management, staff and physicians in acquiring the skills and tools of Adaptive Design in real-time. The LLT takes the lead in the learning and teaching because unit staff and management are generally extremely busy just doing their current work, with little or no space or time for anything else.

The LLT is the initial extra resource necessary to start, but he or she will not stay on the Learning Line. This is not another added "new" position on the unit. The LLT's job is to teach skills and tools that will eliminate ambiguity, assumptions, workarounds and tradeoffs — the first-order problem solving hazards that consume so much time and energy.

Eventually the LLTs will leave to teach other units. By design, each unit's management, staff and physicians use part of that regained time to acquire the skills to increasingly do their own problem solving. As results verify the method, the responsibility for continuing and growing Adaptive Design problem solving becomes management's most important job. One senior manager in a large health system stated it well: "Adaptive Design is not process improvement. It's real-time management development."

I have seen successful LLTs come from many different roles and backgrounds. Clinical experience is helpful, but not essential. These are the key attributes of their success:

- good people skills,
- a desire to learn, and
- a willingness to start with a beginner's mindset.

It is also helpful if the LLTs are known in the organization as trusted and reliable colleagues, folks people have turned to for help in the past. Sometimes management assigns the job to individuals they believe are "on the way up," because LLTs commonly end up knowing more about hospital operations than anyone else!

Along with the LLT, Adaptive Design also requires the appointment of a senior manager to champion the work, act as liaison to the senior team and be the resource for problem solving high in the organization.[11] When the leadership group convenes, it usually becomes quickly obvious which unit would be the best Learning Line. Once the choice is made, the work of knowledge management and learning begin.

Humans learn to walk before they run — after usually much help and many falls. In Adaptive Design, improvement follows "the rules" — in this case, Rule 4: Any improvement must be made in accordance with the Scientific Method, *under the guidance of a teacher*, as close to the patient as possible.

Once the Learning Line is chosen, the LLT, local management and the unit's staff begin to learn under the guidance of a teacher. Initially, this teacher is either an internal or external consultant skilled in Adaptive Design. He or she must be capable of moving the team forward, first by guiding, then assisting, and finally, as skills develop and improve, by increasing local independence.

In conventional consulting, the consultant takes the lead and drives the work. In Adaptive Design consulting, we are there to transfer the adaptive knowledge management skills and tools of Adaptive Design and then develop the "team" through learning-by-doing.[12]

Progressive development of people through problem solving under the guidance of a teacher is fundamental to Adaptive Design and never stops.

---

11 Subsequent to writing this chapter, a powerful tool has been developed to accelerate management learning — the Management Learning Line (MLL). There is more on the MLL in the next chapter.

12 When we refer to a "team," it is always some combination of frontline, teacher/manager and more senior management, as needed, that fits the specific problem being solved. Leadership and management's role in internalizing and growing this capability is the subject of Chapter 10.

Adaptive Design initially makes logical sense to the Learning Line by sharing a fundamental tenet with healthcare: diagnosis before treatment!

The first step in Adaptive Design is to develop a deep understanding of the work ("making a diagnosis") before any changes are made ("initiating treatment"). We diagnose by observing and documenting work on the Learning Line. This creates the Current Condition that shows everyone *this is how we work now.*

Start-up is an important phase for three reasons:

1. Adaptive Design is all about doing. You learn-by-doing. This may seem obvious, but, in reality, moving from the talking phase to the doing phase can be difficult. Someone always wants "more data" or "just one more meeting."
2. The first thing is to observe the work. Through observation, the LLT and management are eliminating assumptions and ambiguity. If they saw it happen, it happened. No questions.
3. As the LLT and management observe and learn, the minds and expectations of the people on the Learning Line start to change.

At the outset, it's not unusual for mindsets on the Learning Line to be negative and pessimistic. I'm sure you can imagine that the moment "a suit" with a clipboard shows up on a unit, red flags wave and alarm bells sound: "Oh no, another efficiency expert to document how I'm not doing my job properly." Or, "I wonder who is going to get laid-off now?" Or, "Here we go again — the next flavor of the month!"

As soon as the LLT and management demonstrate that Adaptive Design is different (i.e., people's ideas are valued, their feelings are important and their development essential), mindsets change. *Clarity, consistency and authenticity* are fundamental to Adaptive Design's success and the old saw is true, "You never get a second chance to make a first impression."

The team members' deportment is critical during this, their first opportunity to establish trust and build optimism among those who will be the learners and, ultimately, the practitioners of Adaptive Design.

The first job of adaptive knowledge management is to learn. Therefore, before even arriving on the unit, we develop a shared understanding among senior management, team leaders and staff that our first job is to learn. Objective number one is to observe and document the work as it really is, not as it is espoused. Nothing more, nothing less. If the consulting team does not "walk the talk," it will not build trust and optimism — it is as simple as that.

To understand the "Current Condition" requires learning new observation and documentation skills. And using the language and framework of the Rules-In-Use simplifies the process of learning. For example, if a cardiac cath lab became the Learning Line, we are guided by and therefore study these elements:

Rule 1 (Activities) — The work of individuals, e.g., RN's, scrub and monitor techs, and cardiologists in the cardiac cath lab;

Rule 2 (Connections) — How one individual adds value to another, e.g., cath lab scrub tech to cardiologist, RN to monitor tech, central supply to RN;

Rule 3 (Pathways) — How many individuals, machines, tools and technology combine to create a complex good or service, e.g., cath lab patient admission through discharge.

Observation starts by exercising authority[13] to make our direction on the Learning Line clear (Ideal Patient Care) and then creating a relationship of "humble learners" to frontline teachers.

From the first hour, we authentically believe (and state openly) that no one knows more about a job than the person doing it. Our team gives the respect these employees deserve for their knowledge and skills. This sense of humility informs the entire effort.

For example, it's not unusual to hear someone on our team say,

> We need your help to move patient care toward Ideal. First, we have to understand how work currently happens. That means you must teach us. No one understands your work better than you, so no one is a better teacher. May we please watch as you do your work so we can learn?

Because observation in the workplace is so fundamental to Adaptive Design, two appendices on the process have been provided at the end of this chapter; one on the essentials of observation and the other on our rules for conducting observations.

Hundreds of people have been taught how to observe safely and effectively, while simultaneously increasing the trust and optimism of staff and management. We've said it before and we'll say it again:

There is no substitute for direct observation.

---

13 Management makes it clear that, although they are there to learn, they are in charge. You can still be in charge and be a "humble learner." For more on the power of authority see Chapter 10.

Documentation

And there is no substitute for documentation of your observations. *"A picture is worth..."* — well, you finish the phrase.

Pictures really do matter. In fact, *no* observation is complete without creating a graphic, pictorial representation of what has been seen. This can be challenging for first-time observers. Simple tools make it natural and easy to learn and, again, the fastest learning comes by doing.

The objectives of documentation are to:

- **Illustrate** what you have seen in the context of where work was done, what was done, who was spoken to and what the discussion was about.
- **Use simple, standard graphics** to facilitate learning. We avoid reports or using written descriptions because, once the skills are acquired, graphical communication is much more effective in teaching and learning.
- Close the loop by **sharing your documentation** with those you have observed. Verify its accuracy with the person who actually did the work, so you honor your learner relationship by checking with the teacher.
- Use every opportunity to continually develop shared understanding by **showing the people doing the work the documentation** and asking for their input.

For example, Figure 1 is the first documentation done by using these methods of the activity of a nurse in one hour on a typical inpatient unit.

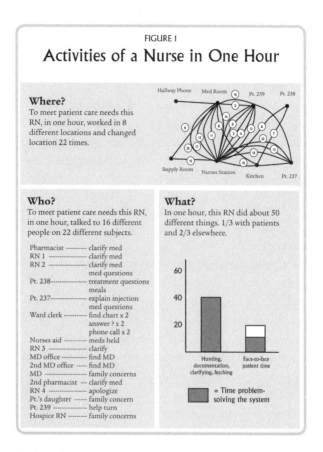

FIGURE I
Activities of a Nurse in One Hour

Where?
To meet patient care needs this RN, in one hour, worked in 8 different locations and changed location 22 times.

Hallway Phone   Med Room   Pt. 239   Pt. 238

Supply Room   Nurses Station   Kitchen   Pt. 237

Who?
To meet patient care needs this RN, in one hour, talked to 16 different people on 22 different subjects.

Pharmacist	clarify med
RN 1	clarify med
RN 2	clarify med
	med questions
Pt. 238	treatment questions
	meals
Pt. 237	explain injection
	med questions
Ward clerk	find chart x 2
	answer ? x 2
	phone call x 2
Nurses aid	meds held
RN 3	clarify
MD office	find MD
2nd MD office	find MD
MD	family concerns
2nd pharmacist	clarify med
RN 4	apologize
Pt.'s daughter	family concern
Pt. 239	help turn
Hospice RN	family concerns

What?
In one hour, this RN did about 50 different things. 1/3 with patients and 2/3 elsewhere.

Hunting, documentation, clarifying, fetching   Face-to-face patient time

■ = Time problem-solving the system

I made this observation at a Boston-area hospital in 1999, but it has been repeated thousands of times by dozens of different observers in a multitude of healthcare environments. Interestingly, as Chapter 8 stated, the approximately 30 percent time in direct patient care documented here is very close to what we continue to see in almost every inpatient environment, now 10 years after the first observation of a nurse.

Execution: An Adaptive Design case study of learning-by-doing.

Several years ago, a 36-bed medical/telemetry unit in a hospital located in the capital city of a large western state became a Learning Line. (This work was documented in an article in *Nursing Economic$*.[14])

---

14 Braaten & Bellhouse. *Improving Patient Care by Making Small Sustainable Changes: A Cardiac Telemetry Unit's Experience.*

It was a particularly difficult time for the hospital. The unit nurse manager had just resigned and the unit was about to undergo a major renovation while the staff would have to move to a temporary location during the construction. Furthermore, for a variety of reasons, some key physicians had lost confidence in the unit and had begun sending their patients elsewhere, even to a nearby competing hospital.

The silver lining in all those clouds was that some unit staff and managers were dissatisfied enough to foster a degree of readiness for change. In particular, they wanted to reestablish physician confidence in their patient care and other hospital departments felt that efforts to improve the unit were long overdue.

A new nurse manager, the nursing director and (significantly!) the hospital's CEO were willing to support applying the principles and practices of Adaptive Design in the unit.

As I have continually reiterated, the first step was to employ direct observation and documentation of the unit workplace. In Adaptive Design, this is called "documenting the Current Condition."

Under the guidance of a team experienced with Adaptive Design, management and staff spent two weeks learning how the work was performed. This learning was grounded in direct observation of activities, connections and pathways throughout the unit and its suppliers. No formal meetings were scheduled, and, as much as possible, no one on the unit was taken away from his or her work.

This documentation resulted in the Current Condition: a detailed representation of the unique realities of work in progress on this unit now. It included the activities of many individuals, important connections, and Material and Information Flows (M&I Flows) over key pathways.

Managers and staff were astonished at the complexity of their work: the surprising number of locations visited in a single hour, the large number of connections made with patients and other staff members and the complexity of the pathways for routine services.

These initial observations served three functions:

1. Managers, staff and physicians discovered that the Adaptive Design team was all about learning, not finding fault or uncovering incompetence.
2. We all learned their work was much more complex and chaotic than anyone had realized.

3. Through their actions and non-judgmental approach, the team began to build trust and optimism among people in the unit.

All three of these outcomes were critical to the success of the undertaking. Once this foundation had been established, the Adaptive Design team was ready to begin creating small changes at the bedside by identifying problems and formulating solutions to test.

Keep in mind that the proverbial North Star guiding this work is Ideal Patient Care. If the system fails to provide Ideal Patient Care, that problem needs to be addressed — now! But moving toward Ideal Patient Care requires thinking and acting differently, i.e., *execution*.

Here's how Adaptive Design provides the missing link: After the Current Condition was completed; everyone discovered that there were lots of problems. So, which to solve first? Should we look for the greatest cost/benefit or do a Pareto Analysis? Or maybe we just "pick the low-hanging fruit," or go for the "biggest bang for the buck."

Actually, none of these techniques were used, and this is where Adaptive Design really starts to change minds and expectations. In Adaptive Design the first problem addressed is *the next problem encountered* in the course of work — and *as soon as it occurs*. This next problem becomes the foundation for immediate problem solving, a fundamental tenet of both the Toyota Production System and Adaptive Design. Problem-solving the next problem that takes place in the workplace is another one of the overlooked secrets of Toyota's success.

In our experience, problem solving in the course of work is very powerful in healthcare. And it usually looks like this: Staff are reminded that the LLTs are there to help them move patient care to Ideal. We state openly that the role of "the system" is to give managers, staff and physicians whatever they need to provide Ideal Patient Care — exactly, customized, immediate, safe, with no waste. So any time that any person does not have what he or she needs, there's a problem to solve *now*.

And how do we know someone does not have what's needed? He will have to signal to a LLT, as in "I have a problem." How long does it take to identify a problem? Once staff members understand they are not just supposed to do a workaround, it takes about a nanosecond to find an employee who does not have what he or she needs to meet patient care needs Ideally.

One staff member quickly signaled that she was missing a special lab specimen bottle recently ordered on the computer. So, what was the first step in solving a problem associated with ordering and delivery of supplies? Yes, you guessed it: direct observation! The LLT carefully watched the process in real-time and then depicted the key elements in a graphic representation of the Current Condition *of this problem.*

Until actually watching supply acquisition in action, all were largely unaware what elements were causing difficulties. From several observations they discovered the process usually involved the following steps:

1. Placing the order.
2. Waiting an unspecified amount of time for the order to be filled.
3. Calling central supply to check on the status of the order.
4. Checking in all the many places where the order might have been delivered.
5. Calling central supply again and describing the product needed.
6. Finally, receiving the product.

How much ambiguity and how many assumptions, workarounds and tradeoffs do you see in this activity? But despite the obvious unwieldiness and unreliability of this process, the staff had lived with it for years. They were just grateful when supplies arrived, on time or not. Changing such unacceptable expectations means changing minds.

What everyone involved quickly learned from the drawing was that the computer-generated order did not contain enough information for the supply technician to know (1) what supply was being ordered, and (2) when it was needed. In other words, lack of specificity was a major culprit, resulting in ambiguity and workarounds.

But this was only a general finding. The next step was to identify the root cause of the problem. This required the problem solvers to analyze the situation and ask specific questions regarding the process. The A3 problem solving tool we introduced in Chapter 7 created a common framework and discipline for their work. Use the A3 format in Figure 2 to follow along and see how these steps fit on an 11 X 17 piece of paper.[15]

To facilitate your learning, I have drawn this A3 on my website at www.johnkenagy.com/book/A3. Log on and you can see Steps I – VI on pages 108 – 111 as if you were drawing the A3 yourself.

---

15 An excellent reference for, and much more complete discussion of, A3's in healthcare is found in Cindy Jimmerson's book, *A3 Problem Solving in Healthcare*, listed in the Bibliography.

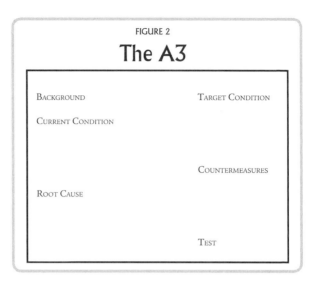

FIGURE 2

The A3

BACKGROUND

TARGET CONDITION

CURRENT CONDITION

COUNTERMEASURES

ROOT CAUSE

TEST

Here's how the analysis advanced (see www.johnkenagy.com/book/A3):

Step I — The **Background** simultaneously frames the problem and creates the business case. *To meet patient care needs Ideally, staff must have the supplies they need when and where they need them. In this case, supplies were not available on time.*

Step II — A graphical, pictorial illustration of the **Current Condition** outlined the specific problem and documented the problem: *a cumbersome, unreliable process that took time away from patient care.*

Step III — Determine the **Root Cause** of the problem to obtain a deeper understanding. During my training by TPS experts, I found they still almost religiously ask "Why?" five times to identify a problem's Root Cause.

This is how it works. Start with the initial problem and ask, "Why did this problem occur?" Then take the answer and ask "Why?" again, repeating the process a total of five times to determine the root cause.

In the following example, the presenting problem was that obtaining supplies (in this case, a specimen bottle) was a cumbersome, unreliable process that took time away from patient care. The Five Why's were:

1. *Why?* The specimen bottle did not arrive when needed.
2. *Why?* Central supply didn't know when the unit needed the specimen bottle.

3. *Why?* The ordering process does not specify the time and place of the supply delivery and what central supply needs to do if the supply order is not clear.

4. *Why?* The connection between central supply and the nurse who needs the supply is not specified (Rule 2).

5. *Why?* ***The entire process necessary to obtain a supply in a timely manner has not been clearly specified.***

Specifying the work becomes easier if you frame the root cause questions using the Rules-In-Use. Most importantly, unlike most conventional quality improvement methods, the Root Cause Analysis is performed *in the workplace*, very close in time and location to the occurrence of the problem. Not in a meeting room, not weeks later, but rather on the floor (now) and with the people who just discovered the problem of this missing supply.

This immediate Root Cause Analysis commonly discloses essential information that is deeply buried in the context of the immediate time and place of this problem. We have found that delaying the Rood Cause Analysis by even a few hours can result in loss of essential information.

The further away in time and place from the problem that the Root Cause Analysis occurs, the more likely that important details will be lost or overlooked.

Step IV — Having identified a Root Cause for this supply problem, the team was now ready to consider solutions. The challenge at this stage was to identify a possible "**Target Condition**" — a hypothesis of a new way to work that eliminates the problem.

Necessary prerequisites for achieving the Target Condition are: (1) Make the approach simple and quick, (2) use current resources and (3) provide the least costly effective solution. Updating or buying a new computer system *would not be an option* under these criteria.

In Adaptive Design, it's always ingenuity first.

In addition, the Target Condition must not cause new problems for others. The key in all problem solving is to have a crystal-clear understanding of the problem's Root Cause — in this case, a lack of specificity regarding the process of ordering supplies. The Target Condition represented graphically and pictorially in the A3, showed a new way to work where the nurse received her supplies when and where she needed them.

Step V — But we don't work that way now. Our work is currently documented in the Current Condition and that caused a problem.

The activities proposed to remedy the problem are called **Countermeasures** — the steps we will take to move from the current problematic work to a targeted, new way to work.

Therefore, creating the Target Condition involved designing the necessary Countermeasures that would specify the timing of the supply order using current resources and without creating new problems.

Using Rule 2 (Every customer-supplier connection must be direct, and there must be an unambiguous yes-or-no way to send requests and receive responses), these Countermeasures would specify the exact time the supplies would be needed, the place of delivery, and importantly, *how* and *who* to signal if the process was not working. Redesigning the supply order was relatively simple, but the hypothesis must be testable. As such, it's essential to know when it does not work. Identifying when the solution fails, not designing a perfect process, is the counterintuitive objective of Adaptive Design.

So, the central supply coordinator (whose name was listed at the nurses' station) was to be notified if the process failed. Creating this feedback loop not only helped improve the unit's experience in ordering supplies, but also made it possible to discover if and when our hypothesis failed. The goal of adaptive knowledge management is to continue to learn, not only on the Learning Line but also for supply chain opportunities throughout the hospital.

Step VI — Most importantly, the Target Condition hypothesis is now testable, verifiable and improvable.

How was it tested? During use, the question was asked, "Yes or No: Are supplies available on time as designed?" If the answer is "Yes," this problem solving effort is completed. If "No," we have to answer the question, "What is it about the way we are working that has created this problem?"

In this case, a clear-cut customer-supplier relationship was established and a testable, verifiable and improvable solution accomplished in the course of work. And it worked!

Engaging staff and management in this type of real-time problem solving yields far-reaching benefits. Most importantly, success imbeds the skills and tools of Adaptive Design into everyday work. The staff quickly discovers that they *can* improve the work. Management learns the value of real-time problem solving and starts to incorporate the skills and tools into their daily work. Increased success builds trust and optimism. Trust and optimism engenders the confidence to do more. Confidence, in turn, creates resilience that allows management and staff to increasingly challenge each other and the status quo.

Moreover, it is safe, because staff and management have experienced a disciplined, structured approach that generates value. That means not only are the individual improvements sustained, the method to continue making improvements is a sustainable part of everyone's work. They only have to keep doing what they now know how to do.

This is how Adaptive Design leads to cycles of increasing returns — the more you do, the more you learn, do, learn, do and... learn!

The doing/learning/doing cycle does not stop, it just gets better. That's Adaptive Design and adaptive knowledge management in action.

The following chart (adapted from Braaten & Bellhouse article) shows a timeline of measurable outcomes that resulted from multitudes of problems solved on this medical/telemetry unit in the course of work. Continued problem solving assured that, not only were the gains sustained, the unit continued to improve. The secret — improvement built into the work of everyone, all the time.

FIGURE 3

Timeline and Measurable Outcomes

OCTOBER 2004
Assess unit's Current Condition:
RN retention is 80%; Productivity is 75%;
patient satisfaction is 3.9 (scale of 1-5).
Unit problem solving begins.

JANUARY 2005
Unit problem solvers trained.

FEBRUARY-MAY 2005
50+ problems solved.
Unit "feels different."

JULY 2005
Retention rate increases to 96%.

OCTOBER 2005
Patient satisfaction increases to 4.8 (scale of 1-5).
Productivity increases to 96%.

JULY 2006
Employee satisfaction increases to 4.03 (scale of 1-5).
A "World Class" designation by surveyors.

It is significant that these results were achieved through a true "grass roots" effort by line staff and managers long after the Adaptive Design LLTs had left and moved on to other units.

This is diametrically different from my past experiences in healthcare, where gains often start to disappear as soon as the consultants leave or the project ends. In a traditional setting, improvements in outcomes are management-driven and often achieved through broad institutional (or system-wide) initiatives.

Moreover, our healthcare culture has tended to reward resourceful employees who, over the years, have learned how to first-order problem-solve by working around the system. Unfortunately, such a combination is a perfect design for eroding gains and improvements, and causing the work to return to its former baseline.

This was brought-home to me at the time I was starting my Visiting Scholar appointment at Harvard Business School. At a Harvard-based healthcare meeting, I ran into a hospital CEO from the healthcare system I had recently left.

We talked about his experience with the latest, "cutting edge" method in process improvement. He summed it up well with this comment: "Yeah, our teams always hit their targets and goals, and everybody celebrates. But the problem is if I don't hold my thumb on that unit, the gains disappear over time."

Healthcare CEOs who want to make a sustainable improvement in their institutions either need lots of thumbs — or Adaptive Design.

In contrast, Figure 3 shows how creating the skills to problem-solve fosters employee optimism, creates cycles of increasing returns, and facilitates sustainable innovation and high performance through new levels of teamwork within individual units and interdepartmentally.

Execution: Building sustainable improvement into the work means changing people's minds.

Adaptive Design discussions commonly lead to questions about "changing the culture." True culture change occurs as staff and management *consistently experience and participate in* a work environment where the goal is to immediately problem-solve toward Ideal.

Here are some examples of how adaptive organizations create environments that shape new behavior by eliminating seven cultural barriers that may be slowing, stalling or stopping sustainable improvement in their organization.

The Seven Cultural Barriers to Sustainable Improvement:

1. Workarounds
2. Fear of Failure
3. Blame
4. Chronic Dysfunctional Behavior
5. Backsliding
6. Lack of Accountability
7. Organizational Silos

1. *Eliminate workaround behaviors by solving "trivial problems."*

Staff quickly learns that there are no "trivial problems." Why? Two reasons: First, since everyone is involved in problem solving as part of everyday work, the resources are available to solve small problems. And, second, "small problems" almost always are bigger than they appear. Remember Toyota's motto, "Solve the small problems close to you and the big problems go away."

For example, in a unit at another hospital, staff had worked long and hard to solve a chronic wheelchair problem. One could never be found, a seemingly trivial problem? But it was not a trivial problem at all. In our initial assessment of the Current Condition, one staff member pointed out that she had worked at the hospital for 20 years and had spent time almost every day looking for wheelchairs. In another 12-hospital health system, they estimated that hunting for missing wheelchairs cost them $500,000 in lost staff time per year.

In this case, after a good deal of experimentation, the staff came up with the elegant solution of creating a "wheelchair parking lot." A specific location on the floor to which chairs would be returned when not in use. This was combined with instructions on the back of the chairs designating the area to which they should be returned: Problem solved? No, not solved completely – but that was okay and actually beneficial. (Read on.)

2. *Decrease the barriers to change by making failure a benefit, not a liability.*

In Adaptive Design, when a solution fails, it's never a failure in the "traditional" sense. Rather, it's an opportunity to learn more and improve again in a structured, disciplined, replicable way.

After the wheelchair system had been in place for a few days, one of our associates arrived on the floor to find a discouraged nurse manager. She had come to work that morning to find wheelchairs scattered around near the elevator, nowhere near the designated parking lot. Her immediate reaction was that others in the hospital just didn't care and were therefore unwilling to help make the new system work.

Aides and transporters had been moving patients the night before, but had apparently ignored the instructions about returning the chairs to the lot. As a result, she was frustrated. If you are experienced in healthcare, you have been in her shoes and shared that feeling. But her negative feelings were short-lived.

The culture of Adaptive Design is to learn from failure. Something about the proposed solution — the way they are currently working — caused this solution to fail. What did that nightshift group not know?

To find out, the nurse manager took a closer look at the instructions on the back of the wheelchairs: *Please Return to 5 West.* That's exactly what the well-intentioned transporters had done! The problem was a lack of specificity about the location of the wheelchair parking lot, not the indifference of other workers. Such self-discovery has the power to break down barriers and create a new sense of unity and shared purpose.

3. *Eliminate blame by proving "it's not people, it's the system."*

The wheelchair problem helped this manager discover and reinforce that Adaptive Design revives quality improvement pioneer W. Edwards Deming's classical principle of focusing on the system, not the people. Every manager should ask herself to what extent the organization is focused on "people problems," rather than "system problems."

This is not to say that every organization is free of people problems, but when given the right tools and the clear objective of achieving Ideal Patient Care, most of those working in healthcare are ready, willing and able to give their all. At least that's been our experience!

The goal of Adaptive Design is to *fix the problem, not fix the blame* on someone else. But individual behavior can be a problem, so we do need an adaptive approach to changing behaviors.

4. *Solve dysfunctional personnel and behavior problems adaptively.*

When personnel behaviors are the issue, Adaptive Design can provide unique and highly objective insights that dramatically alter the character of the interaction with an employee.

This experience occurred on a unit in a mid-sized Mid-Western hospital. The unit manager reported having persistent performance issues with one of the senior staff nurses. This nurse had worked on the unit for a number of years and was well connected in the medical community — both factors that contributed to her sense of entitlement. Numerous one-on-one sessions between the manager and the staff member had not produced any noticeable improvement in her performance.

The ultimate solution proved to be an *adaptive* one. Direct observation of this nurse during the course of work presented a challenge for her to join the entire unit in moving toward Ideal Patient Care. By understanding the nurse's work objectively, the nurse manager was able to frame discussions and problem solving around shared values and de-emphasize the personal angle. As the nurse manager explained:

> I'd literally met with this nurse over 20 times to discuss her attitude. Ultimately, I realized that I don't need to get along with every nurse on my floor to be a good leader; I just need to get them what they need to take care of their patients and have them be part of the solution when they are part of the problem. Adaptive Design has been enormously helpful for making our work more about patients and less about personalities.

When the focus shifted from *"your attitude"* to "caring for *our patients* Ideally," the tone of subsequent discussions changed from performance in general to specific steps this RN could take to help achieve Ideal Patient Care on the unit.

In another case of management resolving a thorny personnel issue, a nursing unit was frustrated by a competent, well-liked nurse who was persistently late for work. Encouragement, reminders, counseling and exhortations had all failed. In fact, the nurse herself was frustrated by her tardiness, but she just couldn't seem to arrive on time.

Finally the manager decided to approach this problem *adaptively*. She had the nurse do self-observation and then specify her morning routine as a Rule 1 Activity. The nurse discovered that her morning routine was designed to fail. She redesigned and timed herself the next morning. With her new morning activities specified, she only had to get up five minutes earlier to be consistently on time. The big change came when she said, "I realize I am not only putting myself at risk by coming late, but it is not fair to my patients or coworkers."

This is a good example of a basic Adaptive Design tenet: The person whose behavior has to change needs to be the person who owns the problem and the solution. As long as it was management's or her coworker's problem and solution, little progress was made despite her good intentions.

Approaching the problem adaptively allowed her to not just own it, but own it safely so she could improve. Even if she arrives late in the future, she knows what she can do to improve — and so do her manager and coworkers.

5. *Eliminate backsliding by repeating what works, relentlessly.*

Remember, Adaptive Design is a skill and skills improve with practice. People who once learn Adaptive Design identify and successfully solve more problems. Success breeds success, so they want to keep problem solving. The most common response from staff and management who have become experienced in Adaptive Design is to say, "I don't want to go back to my old job." Management builds on this natural desire by providing the direction and resources to assure mastery, momentum and stability of real-time problem solving — making it easy to do the right thing.

The ability to change behavior increases because Adaptive Design is a process that builds on itself. Through the initial analysis of the Current Condition, staff begin to trust the method, understand how it works and develop a new appreciation of their work. By gathering first-hand data and information, staff begin to realize the complexity of the tasks they perform on a daily basis and the extent to which the system can thwart their best efforts and those of their colleagues. They quickly come to recognize the forced workarounds and tradeoffs made daily as problems to solve. And **eventually they discover how their behaviors contribute to, and become part of, certain problems that keep the organization from sustaining gains and moving forward.**

As the cartoon character Pogo once said: "We have met the enemy — and he is *us*."

In the case of Adaptive Design, the enemy is not people, but rather the deeply ingrained habits and behaviors produced by years of dealing with ambiguity, assumptions, workarounds and tradeoffs. When people discover the advantages of change, they don't want to go back.

One time, while observing patient registration in the hospice setting, it came to light that patient data had to be entered into the computer system twice. No one asked why — but it didn't take long for the staff members working with Adaptive Design to realize this as taking time away from patients. Soon they asked, "Why are we doing this?"

The goal is to change people's expectations about the work and the systems that are supposed to serve them. Management and staff working adaptively achieve that goal and then improve on it every day.

6. *Create personal accountability by changing minds and expectations.*

Adaptive Design fosters accountability for removing ambiguity, assumptions, workarounds and tradeoffs and then, making it personal.

Consider a nurse who rushes through the hallways of a unit to some place we didn't even know existed for some needed supply in a dark, remote closet. When the nurse is asked how he knew to look there, the answer is invariably: "I've got it all up here in my head." If asked how a new person would know where to find the needed supply, the answer is usually the same: "Oh, they wouldn't."

In a traditionally managed system that knowledge is a point of pride. But in an adaptively managed system, that discovery provides the insight. The metaphorical light bulb goes on and the nurse realizes that this situation is far from Ideal. Then he starts to own the problem, becoming accountable for creating the solution. Personal accountability is much more powerful than enforced accountability and fosters better execution. Remember, execution is the missing link for most organizations and in Adaptive Design, execution is defined as "closing the gap between our goals, aspirations and our current reality."

7. *Break down organizational silos.*

Organizational silos start to disappear as these six previous chronic barriers are progressively removed. Then management and staff discover it is much more productive to bridge silos than maintain walls. It is now part of their culture.

During a return visit to a hospital where we had done some initial work with Adaptive Design, our team found the manager of the emergency department, the pharmacy manager and the manager of the medical-surgical unit gathered around a table using an A3 to solve a system problem that had hindered the delivery of Ideal Patient Care.

It wasn't the kind of interdepartmental "blame game" one sometimes encounters, e.g., no finger pointing, no railing about who did what to whom. Just three experienced managers trying to problem-solve a system failure in a disciplined, structured, "scientific" way.

Execution: Adaptive Design is first about changing minds, then about changing behaviors, and finally about changing systems.

Before long, staff and management recognize that their workarounds and first-order fixes are imbedded in our current system, "just our way" of doing things. Then they discover that solving problems to meet Ideal Patient Care means changing the system because, as in all things, success breeds success. And often unexpectedly! Therefore, Adaptive Design allows staff and management to discover and transform misconceptions that can contribute to underperformance. For example, let's discover and transform, "That problem is too small to worry about. I have bigger fish to fry."

Solve small problems to obtain big — and commonly unexpected — results.

A cardiac chest pain center had complained for years about the inadequacy of drug reference manuals that the pharmacy department was supposed to have fixed. Pharmacy was always "too busy" to focus on such a menial task, so the unit staff were never pleased with the results.

Dissatisfaction is a great Adaptive Design enabler. Using Adaptive Design principles, it became possible for members of the unit to create a team with pharmacy staff, and together they rewrote the manuals. The end product met everybody's needs.

While this is an improvement, it's still not earthshaking. However, the connection with the pharmacy led to further opportunities for improvement and caught the attention of pharmacy management, who asked the hospital's Adaptive Design LLTs to teach them these new problem solving skills.

As a result, one year later this hospital pharmacy reduced their volume adjusted drug costs (VADC) by -2.5 percent, while the VADC increased in the 11 other system hospitals by +11 percent. Total savings: $1.9 million, direct to the bottom line.

Traditional healthcare management says, "It's big solutions for big problems. We don't have time for the small stuff. We have to focus on making the 'big fix.'"

Is that always true? Are there alternatives? What do you think? In my experience, one alternative is: *Create local solutions that can be adapted and rolled out hospital-wide.*

For 11 years, various Do-Not-Resuscitate (DNR) task forces had struggled with trying to develop a clear procedure to alert nursing and medical staff as to which patients should not be resuscitated. Despite the best efforts of many smart and dedicated people (e.g., multiple meetings, resource-consuming task forces and numerous top-down solutions) over that 11-year period, patients continued to be resuscitated against their wishes or those of their family.

This problem solving cycle started on a Learning Line when an RN discovered she had been taking care of a critically ill patient for several hours without knowing that, by his and his family's wishes, he was a DNR patient. Her response — "That's a problem we need to solve."

After observing the process in place, designing an A3 and testing a number of Countermeasures, staff on a Learning Line came up with an experiment involving four signals to staff members:

1. a distinctive red band on the patient's arm,
2. red tape by the patient's name on the unit board,
3. red tape on the outside of the patient's chart, and
4. red tape on the telemetry monitor.

The only glitch in the new system proved to be a procedure for removing the red tape from the patient chart when the patient had passed away or had been discharged. The staff also soon effectively solved this problem.

By testing and validating solutions locally, the hospital increased the likelihood of finding a more general solution. The hospital finance group estimated that unauthorized resuscitations had cost the system at least $65,000 a month in risk management costs. Focusing on making care more Ideal for patients improves performance, including financial performance.

First-order problem solving is not just a frontline malady. How about discovering and transforming a common management malady, "the addiction to fire-fighting and the first-order fix?"

Change a "first-order fix" management culture. Current management methods often mirror the industrial process management model — management finds the solutions, then holds staff accountable.

Initially, working with Adaptive Design can be disconcerting for managers, since it requires a shift in orientation. A manager discovers the opportunity to move from being a "fixer" to becoming an LLT. This means transitioning from being the person called on to put out fires to one who helps staff uncover the root cause of problems and apply the tools and techniques of Adaptive Design in problem solving. Let me repeat, *Adaptive Design is not a fix; it is workplace fitness.*

The power of Adaptive Design results in an overall change in the culture so that problem-solving the system becomes, as one nurse manager observed, "simply the way we work now." This power is very real for those actively doing the work. As Jane RN at St. TAH said succinctly, "We have become intolerant of mediocrity."

I could not have put it better myself.

It has been both enlightening and humbling to recognize that, despite the thousands of hours we have devoted to both learning and teaching Adaptive Design in healthcare, our team has never engineered solutions to workplace problems better than those developed by the staff members on a Learning Line. Their solutions are always more elegant and effective than anything we can imagine.

Why? Because no one understands the work better than those who are doing it.

Appendix One —
Observation Essentials

How and where to start? Ask and answer the following questions:

What is most important?
Patients first. Start all observations as close to the patient (or the end customer in non-patient care areas) as possible.

Where are we going?
Ideal Patient Care sets our direction. Management must make it perfectly clear that the organization is heading toward Ideal. It creates a common strategic purpose and allows the Learning Line to "focus on just one thing." We then conduct observations to discover the Current Condition and its relationship to Ideal.

Why observe people at work?
Two reasons: First, because people are our most important asset. Second, key information is buried in the context of the work that cannot be discovered without direct observation. You can't manage knowledge if you can't discover it.

Where to observe?
Any place work is being done. All work is important.

How will we move care toward Ideal?
Through problem solving by the Scientific Method, which requires a concise understanding of the starting point — the Current Condition.

How do we control for complexity and change?
Simply by first looking for specific problems in real-time. For example, in Adaptive Design, "medication error" is not a problem but an aggregate of thousands of smaller specific problems and system anomalies. Trying to solve medication error is like trying to create world peace — a noble effort but doomed to failure until we can disaggregate the larger issue into its multiple, more manageable, component parts. "I don't have the codeine I need at 2:00 P.M. for Mrs. Jones in room 246." Now that's a problem we can reasonably expect to solve using the Scientific Method.

How can we use the Scientific Method in the work place?
The Scientific Method requires understanding the Current Condition before hypothesizing a better way to work. Because healthcare is so complex and dynamic:

1. The only way to truly know the Current Condition is to see it.
2. To make problem solving "autonomic," the organization must develop the capability to observe the Current Condition continually.

Who should observe?

Observation is a powerful tool for management to use in changing the organization's culture. The tool works in many different ways. For example, management:

- demonstrates that it values the work of individuals by asking permission to observe and be taught,
- creates safety by truly learning rather than by using observation to correct or improve,
- sets the stage to focus continually on the work to generate both professional and business success for the organization,
- starts the transition from a "fault and blame culture" to a scientific systems analysis-based culture, and
- makes it not only safe for local management to observe, but also creates familiarity and welcome for all levels of leadership at the point-of-care.

Appendix Two —
Guidelines to Assure Observations Build Trust and Optimism

Although observations come in many types, they all follow common principles. We will use the example of a detailed observation of the activities of an individual as an example of good observation behaviors.

- Before beginning the observation, brief the person being observed and provide the opportunity for questions about the process.
- Explain any observation forms or materials.
- Let the person(s) being observed know you are there to learn and that they are the teachers. Remind them they are the only ones who truly know what goes on, and that you are not there to critique or evaluate, but rather to learn exactly what happens at the point-of-care.
- If you do not understand what is happening, ask. Here are some safe, non-judgmental, open-ended questions:

  "What are you doing?"
  "How did you know to do that?"
  "When does this usually happen?"
  "Who was that on the phone?"
  "Where did that come from?"
  "How do you know if you are ahead or behind?"
  "When and how would you ask for help?"

- Keep the observation safe: Do not ask "Why?" or, "Why did you do that?" Those questions can imply judgment and you are not there to judge, but to learn.
- Don't correct or offer suggestions or recommendations for improvement unless specifically asked. If there is an immediate patient safety issue (e.g., someone is about to give the wrong medication), alert the person being observed to the problem. Otherwise, observe and honor the opportunity to see real work, not what staff thinks you should see. Your role is to learn how the work is actually done. If staff members suspect you are there to correct or report them, you eliminate the opportunity to be shown actual work.
- To start, don't follow into the patient's room unless asked (or by pre-arrangement). Wait outside the room, observe discreetly and ask what happened. As the observer and staff become more comfortable,

it becomes easier to gain access to the patient's room. In fact, when patients find you are there to learn, they almost always welcome the observation and often are enthusiastic about adding their views of what they need as patients.

- Do the observation as designed: as a testable, improvable Rule 1 Activity.

CHAPTER 10

A NEW WAY OF SEEING: A NEW WAY OF LEADING

"Management is about arranging and telling...
Leadership is about nurturing and enhancing."

– Thomas J. Peters

I n this book's focus on Adaptive Design's power to use knowledge management to develop people, much about management has been implied. Jane RN at St. TAH described how two years before Bill's surgery "management had decided to do something different."

In this final chapter I will pull back the curtain on what management might look like under Adaptive Design: What's the same, what's different?

Management books are full of lists that describe what good managers should do. This book is no exception. Let's examine six great leaders and take an adaptive look at their work.

1. Bill Gates — Microsoft
2. Andrew Grove — Intel
3. William Hewlett and David Packard — the "Bill and Dave" of Hewlett-Packard

4. Herb Kelleher — Southwest Airlines

5. Taichi Ohno — Toyota

In this diverse group of leaders — different industries, different cultures, different backgrounds, different challenges, different management methods, different personalities — one might ask, "What do they have in common?"

First, they were all adaptive in that none had a great idea and just "rolled it out." All became successful through constant learning and adaptation, which led to change, which created success. Secondly, by looking deeper we find they all shared common leadership characteristics.

The Five Characteristics of Successful Adaptive Leaders:

1. Set a clear, consistent, meaningful direction.

2. Develop people as the number one resource.

3. Build trust and optimism.

4. Problem-solve what does not work.

5. Grow opportunistically and relentlessly by challenging the status quo.

Let's examine each characteristic in detail:

1. Set a clear, consistent, meaningful direction for the organization.

People who worked in these organizations in their early stages speak a consistent refrain: "We knew where we were going."

The direction Bill Gates set is legendary: "Get a workstation running our software onto every desk and into every home." That direction led to the greatest accumulation of new wealth in the history of the world.

Sometimes, the direction set at the beginning is less grandiose. For Herb Kelleher at Southwest Airlines it was getting people who typically rode the bus from Dallas to San Antonio to take an airplane instead. Therefore, he focused on just one thing — being the low cost airline. That "disruptive innovation" became the basis for the largest airline in the world, both in number of passengers and in profit.

One myth about change is that people should be able to deal with ambiguity. The fact is that few people deal well with ambiguity and, in healthcare especially, ambiguity is a curse. Staff, physicians and management need to know where they are going collectively, as part of a larger organization.

Great leaders set clear direction in ways meaningful to the people doing work. Remember Jane RN's comment? "We know where we are going!" That is why, in Adaptive design, we constantly talk about Ideal Patient Care. If everyone in your organization does not have a clear, meaningful, purposeful direction tied to their work, the odds are they won't get there.

2. Develop people as the number one resource.

Since four of these leaders developed or led great technology companies, their focus must have been on technology. Right? Wrong! Their great technological success came from trivial technologies.

For example, Bill Gates reportedly bought DOS from Seattle Computer Company for $50,000. Intel reportedly developed their gigantic microprocessor business based on a $60,000 special order from a Japanese calculator company. Hewlett and Packard started in a garage. But they all had one thing in common: Each of these leaders were fanatical about bringing out the best in their people.

It is not cutting edge technology that makes the difference, even in a technology company; it's people. I was describing the characteristics of great adaptive leaders in a grand rounds at Johns Hopkins some years ago. After the presentation, a member of the audience approached me and said something to this effect:

> You have helped me understand something that has always puzzled me. I worked in the early years at Dell. We were designing the latest technology and yet we always worked on old computers, at times, even generations behind what we were developing. Now I understand. We had the technology we needed, but it did not have to be the newest or the best. It just had to do its job. At Dell it was people, not technology, that made the difference.

3. Build trust and optimism.

People make a difference when they work in an environment of trust and optimism.

By all accounts, Toyota's Taichi Ohno was difficult, authoritarian and relentlessly demanding. Stories of his toughness abound. He once told one of his subordinates to "stand right here and don't move until you see the bottleneck in this production line." The implication was he might have to stand there for a week if he couldn't see the problem, but he had learned to trust Ohno's judgment; he was optimistic about success. Eventually he saw the problem he had previously missed. That was the Toyota Way for Ohno.

Bill Hewlett and Dave Packard created the HP Way with a different approach. They went out of their way to be supportive and stay close to employees. They avoided isolated, top-down hierarchies, recognized the achievements of individual employees — HP instituted cash profit-sharing with all employees the year it was founded — and both remained close to employees as HP grew.

Their management was as innovative as their engineering, and their innovations endure: Efficient, no waste organizational structures, bonuses to frontline employees and "management by walking around" have been widely emulated to build trust and optimism in well-run companies throughout the world.

4. Problem-solve what isn't working.

Ideas are important, but none of these companies' successes rested on rolling out a great idea. The ability of these adaptive leaders to take their ideas and relentlessly problem-solve made the difference.

Southwest Airlines, incorporated in 1967 as Air Southwest, originally served just three Texas cities: Dallas, Houston and San Antonio. According to a popular story, the business plan was first sketched out by Herb Kelleher and Rollin King over dinner on the back of a paper napkin. However, a three-year legal battle with entrenched, incumbent airlines kept Southwest grounded until they prevailed in the Texas Supreme Court.

So, not until 1971 did they actually fly an airplane and then not profitably. Continued losses for the next two years plagued the company and, in 1973, they were forced to sell one of their four Boeing 737-200s to Frontier Airlines just to make payroll.

This failure was not the end of the road, however. Their problem solving continued until they discovered how to run a four-plane schedule with three planes! Harnessing the knowledge and creativity of everyone in the organization, they developed many innovations including the "ten-minute turn" that became their standard ground time for years. In 1973, five years after the idea was birthed, Southwest turned their first profit and has done so every year since, a record unmatched by any other airline.

Andy Grove led Intel to become a successful supplier of computer memory through the early '80s. But a seismic change was occurring in the computer industry that destroyed some of the world's greatest firms that could not adapt, including mini-computer maker Digital Equipment Corporation (DEC).

Intel seemed in the same death spiral as profit of $198 Million in 1984 tumbled to $2 million in 1985. That was when Grove and his team famously problem-solved their failing business and transformed Intel from a memory company to a producer of semiconductors and microprocessors. The Pentium chip, the icon and progenitor of much amazing technology, was more than just a great idea. It had its genesis as a solution to a real big problem: failure of their current business model.

Remember, Clay Christensen's research showed it is almost impossible for an established company to innovate into a new business model. The hard facts prove he is correct. But "almost impossible" means some things are still possible. Andy Grove dramatically expanded "the possible" for Intel.

You can expand the possible for your organization. Adaptive Design packages the direction, methods, skills, tools and inspiration that makes "expanding the possible" part of everyone's work, every day.

5. Grow opportunistically and relentlessly by challenging the status quo.

Good managers marshal their forces when an organization stalls. *Great managers opportunistically and relentlessly challenge the status quo by inventing problems to solve — even when everything is working well.* As you'll see later in this chapter, the ability to challenge the status quo (another of Toyota's secrets) lies at the heart of Adaptive Design.

So, those are the "Five Characteristics of Great Adaptive Leaders." That's *what to do.* All management books have lists of what to do. Now I've given you mine. But there is much more to the story.

Next, let's consider the all-important *how* part of the equation: It's everyone's job — leadership and management at the front line!

As frequently happens, a senior executive for one of our clients actually taught us something. She said, "Stop talking about Adaptive Design as 'process improvement.' Adaptive Design is about real-time leadership and management development. And, what is really great, it's imbedded into everyday work!" Clearly, the focus on problem solving to achieve Ideal Patient Care makes leadership and managerial development everybody's job, every day.

In Adaptive Design for healthcare, we always start as close to the patient as possible. Thus far, I have emphasized frontline development, so let's start there and describe the "how" — the work of frontline managers through middle management in an adaptive hospital.

Guidelines and Skills for Adaptive Managers — Front Line to Middle Management

1. Set a clear direction.
2. Support and develop the skill-sets of your team.
3. Develop your team through problem solving.
4. Challenge toward Ideal relentlessly.
5. Move current resources to higher value.

Now let's look at these guidelines in more detail.

1. Set a clear direction.

The need to set a clear direction should not be a surprise. Adaptive Design makes it simple. The manager is accountable for having everyone on the team know that the goal is Ideal Patient Care — exact, customized, immediate, safe, no waste (see Chapter 8).

Jonathan Schechter, Executive Director of The Charture Institute, an innovative non-profit organization based in Jackson Hole, Wyoming, has worked with Adaptive Design principles in an environment that is very different from healthcare: the actual environment. Specifically, The Charture Institute explores issues of growth, change and sustainability in places of ecological and aesthetic significance. In a personal communication Schechter wrote, "A statement of Ideal combines the inspirational and aspirational qualities of a Mission and Value Statement with the practical qualities of a day-to-day managerial tool."

I couldn't say it any better.

Ideal Patient Care should be a part of every orientation for new staff because it immediately establishes a meaningful strategic purpose for their work. New workers discover Ideal is integrated into their everyday work when they signal what they don't have to meet patient needs Ideally.

Managers also learn Ideal is more than a tool for problem solving. I have observed one healthcare manager begin her response to suggestions from staff with, "Well, is it Ideal?" Ideal creates an immediate reference point for individual and team efforts and clearly frames decision-making.

Ideal is the CFO's friend because when someone asks for more resources, managers reframe the question by first asking: "Are we wasting or not utilizing any current resources that could do this job?" Immediately, the issue transitions from "adding more" to, "making better use of" resources.

In visiting adaptive organizations, I see signs describing Ideal Patient Care popping up spontaneously in multiple places: the CEO's office, administrative assistants' desks, unit clerk stations, staff break rooms and physician lounges. Who put them there? Usually, it's the people doing the work. When this happens, obviously the direction is clear and staff are on board.

2. Support and develop the skill-sets of your team.

A manager and all direct reports form an Adaptive Design team, with the manager assuming the role of Learner/Leader/Teacher. Situated particularly close to the frontline, that support includes occasionally assisting team members to first-order problem-solve to ensure patients get what they need.

In Adaptive Design, managers close to the point-of-care do *interruptible administrative work* to accommodate for unpredictable patient demands. For example, a charge nurse might interrupt her work doing scheduling to drop into the point-of-care to cover staff engaged in a cardiac arrest. In turn, the unit manager may need to fill-in temporarily for the now absent charge nurse.

Flexibility is the hallmark of Adaptive Design's success. For this reason, the administrative hierarchy in Adaptive Design — from the frontline to the CEO — is described as the "Help Chain."

In the Help Chain problems rise only as high as necessary. If they can be resolved locally, that is where the problem solving should take place. But if problem solving requires resources that lie at a higher administrative level, the request should move up the chain as quickly as possible. For example, problem solving between two units may need to involve an administrator who oversees both units. This responsiveness creates an administrative Help Chain that extends from the point-of-care to the top of the organization, but which should be used "Just-In-Time" and only as needed.

3. Develop your team through problem solving.

Second-order problem solving is the fundamental real-time development tool, and each manager serves as the Learner/Leader/Teacher (LLT) for his or her team. Then, each layer of the organization acts as the LLT for direct reports, with a primary responsibility for each manager to increase their team members' skill-sets and capabilities.

To develop second-order problem solving, Adaptive Design always starts with problems that are identified by staff during the course of work. The initial problems may seem trivial and self-centered, but every problem solved creates a learning cycle that increases confidence, skills and trust in problem solving and optimism about improving results. These positive attributes, in turn, accelerate the speed of learning. The potential importance of each discovery increases as results build confidence, trust and optimism.

The table below lists the first 10 weeks of experimentation and problem solving by a chest pain diagnostic unit in a Western hospital. Note how the ability to problem-solve developed over time.

Table 1
Chest Pain Unit Problems Solved, First 10 Weeks

1. Small glove par level	11. Integrelin flush
2. Simplify Learning Line	12. Timely Thallium readings
3. Box meals for patients	13. Timely cath lab reports
4. Staff communication	14. Patient discharge education
5. Bradycardia kits	15. Persantine dose availability
6. Cath lab cardiologist block time	16. Nuclear medicine productivity
7. Prioritized patient placement	17. Patient discharge
8. Designated problem-solver	18. Expedited patient check in
9. Drug protocol reference	19. Rapid room turnover
10. Patients ID'ed as DNR	

The first problems solved were relatively simple. For example, small glove par levels and box meals for patients are important, but do not represent great leaps forward. Yet with each experiment, skills and confidence increase, and eventually a problem will develop that dramatically accelerates learning. In this case, it was problem number 5, Bradycardia kits, which offered staff a new, rapid, reliable method to solve a common and important patient care issue.

As you can see, with experience under their belt, the unit's problem solving took-off, making a difference for patients, not only on their own unit but also in connecting units throughout the hospital. How often do you suppose a nursing unit tackles and resolves a thorny problem such as number 6 (an issue involving cardiologist cath lab block time) as part of daily work?

4. Challenge toward Ideal relentlessly.

Every manager will occasionally encounter his or her team not confronting or even recognizing problems. It is then their responsibility to "make a problem" by challenging the workplace. For example: "It takes seven days to get on our orthopedic surgical schedule. How can we use our current resources to make it five?" Or, "We have all this inventory. How can we do our current work and keep less on hand?" Challenging is an important guideline and a *fundamental managerial skill* in Adaptive Design at all levels.

The ability to challenge increases in direct relationship to the trust and optimism generated by successful results. Trust and optimism build resiliency. A resilient unit can tolerate greater challenges.

Ideal Patient Care makes challenging the status quo not only feasible but also relatively simple. As long as managers can identify ambiguity, assumptions, workarounds and tradeoffs (see Chapter 8), they can challenge the work. Then, as the staff becomes increasingly confident, a skilled LLT can up the ante by creating an environment that generates workers who challenge themselves.

I saw an example of this on a medical/surgical unit in a Mid-Western community hospital. They were doing what we call a Focused Learning Event, solving many problems as they occurred, but centered only on a specific larger problem — in this case, optimizing the care of total joint replacement patients. A multitude of important improvements were made, but then the problem solving slowed as staff found fewer problems.

Then the LLT had an inspired idea. She could have simply said, "How can we reduce this inventory?" Instead, she took a different approach. She had each nurse on the unit spend several hours next to a patient, *observing the work from the patient's viewpoint*. Suddenly, a multitude of new problems became obvious as the nurses discovered that while *all may be okay* through their eyes, it's not necessarily so through the patient's eyes. Creating internal challenges is the most powerful challenge of all.

5. Move current resources to higher value.

Problem solving that eliminates ambiguity, assumptions, workarounds and tradeoffs will generate greater value from current resources. As the staff's and manager's work is simplified, and waste, rework and redundancy are eliminated, personnel can increase their productivity without working harder. Therefore, they are available to move to higher valued work.

Management is accountable to realize this advantage for the organization. As such, it's a good problem to solve.

For example, the Current Condition at the outset of our work on a medical/surgical inpatient unit showed nurses spending about 23 percent of their time in direct patient care. After 13 months of problem solving, nurse involvement in direct patient care increased by 135 percent to 54 percent of a nurse's time. More than half of nursing work was now spent directly in patient care.

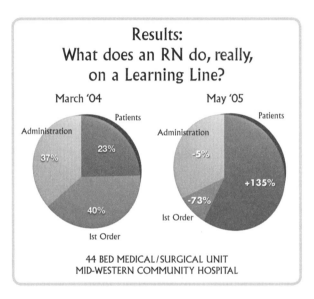

Where did the gains come from? Rather than push for more nursing time at the bedside, Adaptive Design eliminated the first-order problem solving (in this case, a 73 percent decrease) and administrative time (5 percent decrease) that keeps nurses away from the bedside. Thus, they become more productive in patient care.

With Adaptive Design, productivity *will* increase. In our experience, it is automatic. Capturing that value is a fundamental role of management. Increasing productivity in Adaptive Design generates economic value not by layoffs, but by redirecting work to higher value.

For example, this nursing unit eventually redirected some of the work of 12 nurses and a nurse educator into facilitating problem solving. The result was more than 330 problems solved in 13 months that increased the unit's throughput and productivity (14 percent increase), while lowering length of stay (8 percent decrease). At the same time, they had the greatest increase in patient satisfaction in a 17-hospital system. The financial result was $1,700,000 in cost savings and new revenue. That is the essence of Adaptive Design: create more with less by eliminating problems that clog the system with waste, rework and redundancy.

The lesson to take home is this: Do not make improvement a project or special event, but rather part of everyone's work all the time. These examples demonstrate how management can focus on developing and supporting problem solving to get patients what they need *Ideally*. When that happens, work transitions from a "meeting focus" to a "frontline focus." This mirrors Toyota's managerial "shop floor focus."

How does the mindset of upper management change? What about the work of senior managers? The guidelines are the same; however, the order, emphasis and refinement of the skills change. In particular, **moving current resources to higher value** takes on increasing importance the further up you go in the organization.

Adaptive guidelines and skills for senior management, in order of importance:

1. Set direction.
2. Move current resources to higher value.
3. Challenge toward Ideal relentlessly.
4. Support and develop adaptive skills and tools throughout the organization.
5. Facilitate problem solving.

Just as on the frontline, *setting a clear direction* is Guideline #1. At the start, a CEO or COO must be perfectly clear about where the Learning Line (and eventually the organization) is going. Ideal sets the framework and provides the orientating North Star that guides the change in the status quo and conventional thinking.

Moving current resources to higher value then becomes Guideline #2. Establishing a Learning Line and problem solving in the course of work begins the cycle. But habits and behaviors by the senior team can also be part of the problem.

For example, one of the most difficult challenges in setting up a Learning Line is to have the organization *stop spending more money* on the Line. The goal is to use Ideal and immediate problem solving to decide what to do in a scientific, testable, verifiable and improvable way. You cannot do good science without a stable baseline so, at the beginning, we ask that management *not* initiate new projects, buy new technology and hire more consultants on the Learning Line. In other words, don't spend more money!

Even in cash-strapped organizations, you would be surprised how difficult it is to stop *buying* the solutions and start developing current assets and resources to their highest value.

Adaptive Design quickly becomes a friend for CFOs who are inundated and beleaguered by a multitude of capital requests. For example, in a maturing Adaptive Design organization, *buying new solutions or adding resources should never be an option* as long as workarounds, tradeoffs, waste, rework and redundancy can be eliminated.

Guideline #3, *Challenging toward Ideal,* is a powerful way to reorient organizations from the habit of buying solutions to the habit of finding solutions. An outpatient surgery unit using Adaptive Design was scheduled to have three new computerized medication dispensing machines installed. The vendor said this was "best practice" based on the size of the unit.

The COO challenged the director of the outpatient surgery unit on this recommendation, and the challenge was accepted by the director who had trust and optimism in the unit's problem solving capability. Experience with Adaptive Design provided her with opportunities to solve problems and eliminate waste locally. The staff and frontline management rose to the challenge and redesigned their work to eventually eliminate the need for two of the three machines.

New capital requests should always be challenged on the basis of eliminating waste or moving current resources to higher value. Challenging is a very big part of senior management's role and, by fulfilling it, the whole organization moves forward.

The last two guidelines create new capability because they run counter to long-standing, conventional management practices.

	CONVENTIONAL MANAGEMENT	ADAPTIVE DESIGN
GUIDELINE 4 Support & develop adaptive skills	Gather and move information to decision makers. The bigger the decision, the higher it goes. Aggregate problems and implement big solutions using consultants and technology.	Develop and coordinate decision rights moved close to information. Disaggregate problems. Problem-solve to develop local skills and ingenuity. Challenge to create accountability.
GUIDELINE 5 Facilitate problem solving	Management, committees, teams, taskforces, consultants and technology implement big solutions and hold people accountable.	Develop resources and use new skills to solve problems as close to the patient as possible, using only the resources needed.

Organizations make this transition by testing and validating Adaptive Design and then generating results. Establishing a frontline Learning Line allows a senior team to completely test and validate every aspect of Adaptive Design — at low risk. Learning Lines **always** produce and out-perform. Here are some results from Adaptive Design units:

Surgical Productivity and Compliance:

- Increased surgical volume 16 percent,
- While decreasing surgical staff overtime 14 percent,
- 95 percent JCAHO compliant.

The combination of increasing volume while simultaneously decreasing overtime and increasing JCAHO compliance is a perfect example of the power of real-time improvement based in the work. The key to this kind of success is to not implement projects focused on throughput, overtime or JCAHO. For example, you'll hit your volume targets, but miss the small tradeoffs and workarounds that silently increase overtime or decrease safety. This operating room focused on just one thing (Ideal Patient Care), and did one thing (immediate problem solving when work was not Ideal). They solved the small problems close to them and the big problems went away.

Supply Chain Performance:

The supply chain is a natural for Adaptive Design. Here are examples from two different supply chain Learning Lines. The key to these results in each institution was a materials/supply chain manager who committed to using Adaptive Design to solve problems as they happened.

HOSPITAL SUPPLY CHAIN LEARNING LINE CONNECTED TO A SPECIFIC UNIT		
	Before Adaptive Design	With Adaptive Design
Evaluate unit supply room for restocking	30 minutes	2 minutes
Retrieve items from warehouse	25 minutes	10 minutes
Restock unit supply room	15 minutes	3 minutes
Days restocking done/week	3 days/week	7 days/week
Total restocking time/week	210 minutes/week	105 minutes/week

HOSPITAL SUPPLY CHAIN LEARNING LINE FOCUSED ON THE WAREHOUSE		
	Before Adaptive Design	With Adaptive Design
Pick path	249 ft.	120 ft.
Pick times	47 minutes/order	23 minutes/order
Receiving	8 hours	6.5 hours
Departments serviced	12 serviced in 9 hours	23 serviced in 9 hours
Annual inventory turns	23	42
Inventory days on hand	15	8
Time saved		4 man-hours/day
Floor space savings		1320 sq. ft.
Productivity increase		5%
FTE savings		.9 FTE (moved to higher value work)
Reduced warehouse inventory		-30%

These were not one-time results. Each of these managers has continued to problem-solve their supply chain systems and each has improved on these numbers. How? Improvement is just part of the work!

Retention and Recruitment:

- 51 percent decrease in staff turnover,
- Highest staff engagement scores (12-hospital system) for 3 consecutive years.

A huge, hidden cost in healthcare is the cost of replacing staff. One hospital estimated the cost to replace one nurse at $35,000. Adaptive Design depends on building trust, optimism, high performance and innovation. Not only does that create a better environment for patients, it automatically creates a better, higher valued environment for staff and physicians.

The Learning Line gives the frontline an opportunity to develop new habits, behaviors and methods in a knowledge-management, constant-improvement mode. Until recently, the frontline has had an advantage over the senior management team because senior teams have not had similar opportunities to test and validate Adaptive Design as a strategy and leadership method in their work.

Just as I finish writing this book, we are testing the solution to that problem with the introduction of the Management Learning Line (MLL) in two health systems. The MLL focuses on enabling management to use Adaptive Design's knowledge management capability strategically to accelerate gains for the whole organization. It is the Management Learning Line that ultimately takes the lead in designing and creating the business and care model innovations that Adaptive Design enables.

The challenge for senior management is familiar: constant firefighting and the Recurrent Major Initiative Syndrome mentioned in Chapter 8. This often leads to a continuous flurry of activity that appears productive while, in fact, is creating roadblocks to execution of essential strategies for success.

I remember my experience as an executive with the syndrome and how it affected me. It felt much like what my Nebraska farmer aunt used to tell me, "Boy, you are like a pig on ice; you are moving really fast, but you aren't going anywhere."

As we have mentioned many times before, Adaptive Design is simple, but not easy. The goal of the Management Learning Line is to take key leaders off the problem solving/multiple initiative treadmill and give them the opportunity to revitalize, regain their authority and lead more effectively.

The MLL focuses on moving the organization from left to right on the chart below. In making the move, the current top-down approach transforms to an adaptive knowledge management framework.

	CURRENT	ADAPTIVE
What?	Big problems, big solutions. Best practice, consultants and technology. **Knowledge outside**	Solve small problems by rapid, local experimentation and learning. **Knowledge inside**
Who?	Management, committees, taskforces, consultants, experts. Big expensive solutions decided on high in the organization	Everyone, but using only the resources needed to solve "this problem now"
How?	Gather data; analyze, plan and predict; implement, monitor and hold accountable	Management creates and challenges, disciplined, structured real-time problem solving
Where?	Meeting rooms	As close to the problem as possible
When?	Weeks, months, years	Hours, days, weeks
Why?	Hit targets and goals, profitability, compliance, lower costs	Ideal Patient Care, develop people to continuously improve

Stay tuned for more results from our MLL experience and learning.[16]

It may seem surprising that in a method based on problem solving, the last guideline for senior management is problem solving. But, on reflection, the explanation is obvious. The entire organization below the senior management team is focused on problem solving.

The more senior the manager, the more his or her focus should be on building problem solving capability, not solving problems. Remember: "Solve the small problems close to the work and the big problems go away."

Metaphorically, the management system is like the brain and nervous system of the human body. Senior management sets direction, anticipates problems, protects the organization from threats and establishes order and cohesion throughout the system. As such, they are the "brains."

But a brain can't stop to think about all the actions and activities necessary to keep our body functioning, like accelerating the heart rate for exertion, fine tuning temperature control or extracting energy from oxygen or food. For that, we depend on another system — the autonomic nervous system — to create the feedback loops and control functions that keep a complex human body in action.

This metaphor illustrates Adaptive Design in two unique ways. First, Adaptive Design develops and greatly increases the power of the organiza-

---

16 Based on my recent experience, I believe the Management Learning Line will become the key accelerator of adaptive innovation within established organizations. Visit JohnKenagy.com for up-to-date information on adaptive management. It is the new frontier for healthcare learning and improvement.

tion's "autonomic nervous system" to respond locally to unexpected changes in the environment. You don't have to stop and think about it, it just happens. That's the power of solving problems with real-time, second-order, systemic solutions as close to the problem as possible — and with only the resources needed to solve the problem now.

Secondly, Adaptive Design expands the brains of an organization, and here's how: As many of you who practice Lean know, Toyota, early in its development, identified the Seven Wastes: defects, inventory, over-processing, waiting, motion, transportation and overproduction.

And now, in its subsequent development as an adaptive knowledge management company, it has identified the 8th waste, the "greatest waste of all." This is the waste of a human brain — not developing *and not using* the cognitive capacity of every employee. Again, the greatest waste of all!

In the *Fast Company* article, "No Satisfaction at Toyota," written by Charles Fishman (2007), Fishman points out that one of the subtle but distinctive characteristics of a Toyota factory is that the supervisors and managers are not bosses, in any traditional sense. "Their job is to find ways to do the work better, more efficiently, more effectively." For example, Fishman describes a Toyota plant as less a factory and more "a really big brain — a kind of laboratory focused on a single mission: not how to make cars, but how to make cars better."

Imagine how your own institution might be transformed as one really big brain, single-mindedly focused on providing Ideal Patient Care.

Management cannot be on top of everything in health care in the traditional "top-down" sense. It's just a fact of life in the everyday work of our complex business that no healthcare manager or executive can be on every floor, in every lab, in each exam room, 24 hours a day, 7 days a week, 365 days a year.

At Toyota and in Lean processes and tools, the Japanese phrase of *genchi genbutsu* translated as "go to the spot," is a basic tenet of the work. The lesson is that management must go at times to the work to learn. There is no doubt that that is true.

But the problem is healthcare is much too complex, dynamic, and unpredictable for every manager and every executive to watch and think about even the specifics of their area of responsibility, let alone a whole organization. "Management by walking around" is a nice idea, but too often, in my experience, it is more "walking around" and much less "management."

Therefore, Adaptive Design recruits the eyes and trains the brains of *every person* in the organization to identify and respond to problems in the course of everyday work, as problems arise. A CEO may be responsible for the work of thousands of people, but, in an adaptive work culture, he or she can rest easy at night. *Everyone* is watching. And everyone is thinking. *Everyone is genchi genbutsu.*

Here's a Toyota knowledge-management example of creating and training brains taken from my experience. As part of my training, I had the opportunity to observe TPS expert Hajime Ohba at work. Mr. Ohba (as everyone knew him) was the head of the Toyota Supplier Support Center (TSSC), which made him, at that time, the "Grand Guru" for the Toyota Production System in North America.

Visiting a manufacturing facility that his team was consulting with, Mr. Ohba was on the shop floor being presented the work in progress. As I observed, a TSSC consultant was describing the results of an experiment to improve the changeover time of a key piece of equipment. ("Changeover time" is the amount of time it takes to convert a machine from making one part to making a similar part of a different size or type.) The consultant proudly presented how her team had dramatically improved changeover time by 50 percent, very close to their predicted 60 percent.

Expecting congratulations, the consultant was instead greeted by a series of questions from Mr. Ohba:

- Did you consider eliminating this step?
- Could you have used two screws instead of three?
- Could you reposition supplies to make them easier to access?

Then Mr. Ohba smiled, gave the consultant a pat on the back and walked away to the next station.

I was puzzled by Mr. Ohba's response. How could he not offer congratulations for such a dramatic improvement? Later it dawned on me. *It wasn't the result that made the difference, it was the rigor and the learning, the Scientific Method that was important to Ohba.*

He wanted the consultant to question why she had made the prediction of a 60 percent improvement in the first place. What was it about the work that she and her team did not understand that led to unexpected results — the 50 percent improvement rather than the predicted 60 percent? What was the flaw in their hypothesis? What aspects of the work had the team failed to understand? What more could they have discovered?

Remember Chapter 7's Rule 4: **Any improvement must be made in accordance with** *the Scientific Method,* **under the guidance of a teacher, as close to the patient as possible.**

A true scientific experiment has a high level of specificity as to method and expected result. Mr. Ohba believed that his TPS consultant should have had a much more precise idea of what possibly could be changed, and the exact amount of time that she anticipated saving in the production cycle as a result of the modification. The 50 percent reduction in turnover time was a positive outcome, but she and her team had expected 60 percent, and that means additional inquiry was needed; there was still opportunity for deeper learning and greater improvement.

Mr. Ohba also demonstrated the essence of *genchi genbutsu.* He was not "managing by walking around." He "went to the spot" as his own specified Activity (Rule 1) with a testable, verifiable, improvable objective: what could he learn about this team's performance and how could he challenge and improve it.

He was also demonstrating with clarity, consistency and authenticity that *in every failure or unexpected result lies a hidden opportunity.* That's adaptive knowledge management to the nth degree. Toyota has been developing and nurturing this capability for 50 years; I don't expect healthcare to jump magically to this level of excellence. But healthcare should definitely start, and Adaptive Design is the proven method that makes it happen.

Changing people's minds is the essence of adaptive knowledge management. Mr. Fujio Cho, former Chairman of the Board of Toyota was quoted as saying, "No mere process can turn a poor performer into a star. Rather, you have to address employees' fundamental way of thinking." Adaptive Design changes people's minds about what they can achieve individually and collectively.

Given Toyota's focus, experience and effectiveness in the development and empowerment of people, do you think General Motors' traditional, data-up/implement down, industrial mindset ever had a chance to win the competitive battle? First, minds need to be changed. That's disruptive innovation!

Mr. Ohba, The Five Managerial Guidelines and a Healthcare CEO

Mr. Ohba's *genchi genbutsu* example also helps illustrate the Senior Leadership Guidelines in an adaptive organization:

1. **Set direction** — This has obviously already been accomplished. All on the team improving machine changeover knew they were heading for manufacturing Ideal, so there was no hesitation or wavering on Mr. Ohba's part to challenge.

2. **Move current resources to higher value** — The machine's turnover time will almost surely be improved because of his questioning, but more importantly, the human resources will be better prepared to deliver higher value.

3. **Challenge** — How did he achieve 2 and 3 above? By challenging the expected status quo. How could he so bluntly challenge and then just walk away? Over time, a clear direction, a stable, disciplined problem solving method and past success have built trust and optimism in this team. Trust and optimism builds resilience. Resilient teams can be challenged. The more resilient the team, the tougher the challenges it can face.

4. **Support and Develop** — Mr. Ohba used this problem solving event to further develop the skills of this team.

5. **Facilitate problem solving** — Notice that he did not solve the changeover problem, but rather challenged the team to do so. He just walked away, demonstrating he was not there to provide the answer, but to ask hard questions. The messages are clear — management provides the support and the challenge; the frontline provides the answers over and over again.

Here is a healthcare example of a hospital CEO following these guidelines: Sarah Jones (not her real name) makes it clear that her organization is heading toward Ideal and then plans rounds to learn of recent problem solving on a specific unit.

Her rounds only take about 10 – 15 minutes but, importantly, are designed as a Rule 1 Activity with her testable outcomes in mind. The staff or manager doing the work presents the problem in the context of an A3. The staff's accomplishment is honored by Sarah's presence, while she gains deep and significant insights into current frontline work.

She also has a unique opportunity to question, inquire and challenge by bringing her breadth of view of the entire organization to this unit. That adds an important perspective to their work. She reinforces the organization's strategic direction by asking, "How does this work take us closer to Ideal?" Her last question, closing the rounds, is almost always the same, "So what did you learn?" Sarah says *she* learns more than the staff from her rounds.

That's a great example of an adaptive leader: simple, direct, focused, specified by the Rules and adding value. And that's *genchi genbutsu*.

The extent to which this notion of continuous learning in pursuit of constant improvement is part of the Toyota culture is described in Fishman's 2007 Fast Company article I quoted earlier. Says Fishman:

> Toyota's competitiveness is quiet, internal, and self-critical. It is rooted in an institutional obsession with improvement that Toyota managers instill in each one of its workers, a pervasive lack of complacency with whatever was accomplished yesterday.

Through our work with Adaptive Design, we have seen the extent to which this approach can change the work culture in healthcare and can lead to an increasing intolerance of anything less than Ideal for each, individual patient.

One of my most rewarding learning experiences occurred while I was observing a very accomplished Adaptive Design medical/surgical unit in a large Mid-Western hospital. This unit created three nurse LLTs to facilitate problem solving by eliminating less value-added work from their daily routines.

As I walked on the unit, I discovered all three of the nurses engaged in an animated discussion over several A3s. I asked another nurse, "What are they so excited about?"

She answered, "They are going over all their A3s that *failed*. You can't imagine all the cool things they have discovered."

Developing that kind of competence, energy and commitment requires changing peoples' minds. Currently, most healthcare managers and executives focus on gathering more data to find more solutions.

The problem with such "top-down" approaches is that they promote a passive orientation to change in the workplace ("It's somebody else's job"), and could lead to a response at the point-of-care that can be sluggish, apathetic ("This too shall pass") or, worse yet, antagonistic ("I can ignore or refuse").

In Adaptive Design, management's focus transitions from finding solutions to leading people and developing their knowledge, creativity and problem solving ability in an exceptionally disciplined, structured way, always focusing on meeting patient care needs Ideally. It is very much a change of mindset.

We have found this change of mindset occurs in every unit that has developed Adaptive Design problem solving as a routine in the course of work. But it does not happen overnight, nor does it mean some parts of the team do not remain entrenched in more traditional management approaches. In addition, because Adaptive Design starts and grows locally and is quietly embedded into everyday work, it is possible for management to miss opportunities to use it. No big projects, no big meetings, no big capital investments — that's all good, but it does lower Adaptive design's visibility in the eyes of management not directly involved.

For example, one hospital in a large 17-hospital health system had skilled Learner/Leader/Teachers, a successful Learning Line from surgery through an inpatient medical/surgical unit and had used Adaptive Design to generate significant savings and efficiencies in the supply chain. But when faced with a huge investment in an electronic medical record (EMR), the corporate office took a much more traditional, consultant and expert-driven, big project, top-down, design/implement approach to system roll-out. They thought traditionally, not adaptively, because their mindset had not had the chance to change.

The results in the first hospital go-live were disappointing. Not only was the project behind schedule and over-budget, nursing productivity fell significantly and it took nine months for RN's and LPN's to be able to return to their pre go-live patient loads.

But some managers in this hospital system had had a change of mindset because of their Adaptive Design experience. Therefore, there was an alternative to just "trying harder" on the next go-live. People within the system raised a red flag, challenged the status quo and asked the questions, "Could we use Adaptive Design to better prepare staff for the new EMR system? Could Adaptive Design facilitate problem solving post go-live? Could that improve our results?"

The EMR system management agreed to accept the challenge and decided to test using Adaptive Design to prepare for the next hospital go-live. This time the results were significantly different.

Hospital staff in the Adaptive Design-prepared hospital were able to care for a full patient assignment in just two months, a 78 percent improvement from the previous go-live with a savings to the system in reduced overtime, agency nursing and additional revenue in increased throughput estimated to be $9 million, much of which was direct to the bottom line.[17]

The system vice president in charge of the EMR rollout was quite succinct in her assessment, "Skills training in Adaptive Design is as important or more important than any [EMR] changes that may occur." It's people, not the technology, that really makes a difference. Now that's a change in mindset.

When the focus in on Ideal Patient Care and improvement is everyone's work — every day — positive results follow. In Adaptive Design, management, staff and physicians look at their work with changed minds. But since the work is learn-by-doing, the change in mindset only goes as far as the people who have experience using Adaptive Design.

Therefore, adaptive management is challenged to use all the characteristics of great adaptive leaders mentioned at the beginning of this chapter — particularly the admonition to grow Adaptive Design capability by "opportunistically and relentlessly challenging the status quo."

For example, in Adaptive Design, quality is not a department and improvement is not a project. Furthermore, making a difference for patients is not someone else's job. Quality, safety, productivity and improvement — moving patient care toward Ideal — is everyone's responsibility, all the time.

But the status quo thinking in most organizations at the frontline and in traditional management is the opposite. Therefore, adaptive management needs to continually, opportunistically and relentlessly challenge that kind of status quo thinking. It takes a combination of empowerment and authority. Adaptive Design management empowers people with this unstoppable desire to learn. In turn, and essential to increasing empowerment, Adaptive Design develops and increases the authority power of leadership to challenge the status quo.

In traditionally managed organizations, empowerment and authority are rarely mentioned in the same breath. This chapter on leadership closes with a commentary on how these two seemingly disparate attributes are inextricably linked.

---

17 These and other Adaptive Design savings were documented in the as yet unpublished paper, listed in the Bibliography, *Workflows & the Electronic Health Record: Applying Toyota Principles to Improve Implementation*. Please contact me at John@JohnKenagy.com if you would like to see the full paper.

Empowerment

Many management books talk about empowering employees. It has become almost a cliché that "great leaders empower their people." The reality is, however, that empowerment often means taking power away from some people and giving it to others; unfortunately, this "power transfer" is often unstable, temporary or ineffectual. Nothing really changes.

Adaptive Design is empowering to employees, since decisions formerly done by managers are now done much closer to the work. Employees can problem-solve and change a "best practice" — that's power.

But there is no transfer of power. *Instead there is a net increase in power at all levels of the organization.* This happens as management transitions from moving information up, to directing and coordinating decision rights that are moved to where the information resides: in the workplace. The increase in power is generated because Adaptive Design is specific about *matching accountability with control.*

All managers are familiar with the common problem of being held accountable for work over which they have no control. CEOs are supposed to be accountable for safety in their hospitals, but the nature of healthcare puts the safety of an individual patient completely outside the CEO's control. Managers in every system where we have worked are routinely held accountable for work over which they actually have little or no control. This discrepancy is built into the nature of a traditional, industrial-style top-down system and is rarely even questioned.

In turn, we have all seen situations in which individuals have control over actions for which they cannot be held accountable. Physicians have complete control over the legibility of their handwriting, but, in my past 37 years, I have never seen even one organization that could hold physicians accountable for legible handwriting.

Adaptive Design solves this problem by tightly linking accountability and control. That generates increased power at all levels: frontline, middle management and senior leadership. Here's how: Adaptive Design empowers frontline staff to change standardized work, even best practices, that fail to meet patient needs *Ideally*. That is a lot of power. But *they are simultaneously held accountable* to follow a disciplined, structured methodology to make that change "using the Scientific Method under the guidance of a teacher."

By definition, if the solution creates problems elsewhere, uses unnecessary resources or fails to resolve the problem, *it is another problem to solve.*

Therefore, the accountability to redesign the solution is built into the work. This feedback loop, inherent in the structured problem solving method, assures that accountability and control are closely linked.

Problem solving in Adaptive Design is not an *ad hoc* event carried out by people working by their memory of past experiences. It is done under a clear, simple, consistent and pervasive set of rules. Remember Jane RN's comment at St. TAHs, that,

> [A]nother unexpected discovery was that, to improve, we all had to follow certain rules. At first, based on our past experience, everyone was afraid of more rules. But soon we discovered that the rules made it easier and safer to learn and improve.

Returning to the brain and nervous system metaphor, Adaptive Design is much like the natural physiologic feedback loops present in the human body. Our brains can't stop to think about constantly fine-tuning to our environment. So we depend on an autonomic nervous system working underneath our consciousness to manage all these essential details. The autonomic system functions because physiologic rules and feedback systems are always modulating our body's response to a constantly changing environment.

Adaptive Design empowers an organizational "autonomic nervous system" that uses rules, feedback and accountability to modulate the response of the organization to its ever-changing environment. In fact, Adaptive Design creates *autonomic innovation*; you don't have to think about it, it just happens.

Management matches accountability to control through the Rules. By directing, coordinating and challenging decision rights moved to where the information is (i.e., in the workplace) the management "brain" is now free for essential activities it needs to accomplish. Adaptive Design defines these senior leadership activities based on the natural power of authority in human societies.

In my own experience as a healthcare executive, going to meetings, fire-fighting and the Recurrent Major Initiative Syndrome actually worked to subvert my authority. The role of authority is a powerful attribute of Adaptive Design. Today, I see healthcare management with new opportunities to develop and exert authority in a positive way.

The Power of Authority in Adaptive Design

Authority has taken a tough rap lately. Authority was a scourge and a curse for many of us who lived through the infamous flower-child '60s and

'70s. Most from that generation express a concern or fear of authority; it is something we want to avoid.

In actuality, authority is an essential human attribute that allows us to work together in coordinated ways for common benefit. Humans, as social animals, have built-in respect for authority. It is part of our DNA. Our human expectations honor the power of authority, particularly when we are in trouble.

Think about it. When in trouble, we look to our leaders (organizational, political, religious, familial) for help. We grant power to authority because we expect authority to help us. Ronald A. Heifetz, M.D., at the Kennedy School of Government at Harvard, presented this concept of authority power in his 1994 book, *Leadership Without Easy Answers*. I had the good fortune to study in his learning laboratory class at the Kennedy School.

As you will see below, Heifetz lists three specific powers of authority. Through my experience with Adaptive Design, I have added a fourth:

1. We give authority the power to **set direction**. When in trouble, we expect authority to tell us where we need to go. We need direction, a common purpose to work together collectively. We also expect authority to inspire us to reach beyond ourselves. As I speak to many people who worked in great adaptive organizations (as noted at the start of this chapter), they always say, "We knew where we were going!"

2. We give authority the power to **protect** — and we expect that protection. Great leaders let people feel safe about challenging the status quo, testing procedures and discovering new methods. They vigilantly scan for and defuse potential threats. And finally, we give them the power to mobilize and redirect resources in response to threats. Whether a successful teacher, vigilant policeman or an experienced general, we expect protection and grant effective leaders the authority power to provide it.

3. We grant authority the power to **create order**. "Help us work together effectively." We anticipate, in times of trouble, to be orientated to our places and roles. We expect authority to control internal conflict and to remove barriers to success. Finally, authority helps us establish methods and norms of behavior for our common good. In his popular book, *Good to Great*, Jim Collins identified *structure* and *discipline* as two key characteristics of greatness. Great organizations thrive on order.

4. Adaptive Design adds a fourth power of authority: The power to choose the method of **decision-making**. There are many ways in which individuals and groups make decisions. For example:

- Autocratic (Do it!)
- Technical (Find the expert.)
- Democratic (Let's vote.)
- Consensual (We'd better all agree.)
- Adaptive (Together let's test and problem-solve how to change.)

Each of these decision-making methods is important. The key is to appropriately match the method to the problem. Effective use of authority requires exercising these four powers appropriately. Here's how Adaptive Design guides and empowers authority.

Authority power resides at all levels of the organization, but the greatest formal authority lies with the senior management team. Unfortunately, senior managers are often so busy fighting fires and going to crisis meetings that they have little time to exercise their authority.

Under Adaptive Design, "solve the small problems close to you and the big problems go away."

By moving problem solving into the workplace and developing the knowledge, creativity and problem solving ability of everyone in the organization, the big problems start to vanish. This frees senior management to pursue its natural leadership role. And what is that role? To establish authority within the organization through the following:

- Direction — "We are heading toward Ideal Patient Care."
- Protection — "You are safe to challenge the status quo by signaling problems when care is not Ideal."
- Order — "We work this way: disciplined, structured, replicable, testable, verifiable and improvable problem solving as close to the patient as possible. We follow the Rules."
- Decision-making — "There are times for autocratic decisions, democratic decisions, technical decisions, etc. But when facing an adaptive problem, we use adaptive decision-making."

Table 6 compares three decision-making methods — technical, complex technical and adaptive. If it's a technical problem, find the expert and solve it. But if it is an adaptive problem, technical solutions are designed to fail.

Table 6

Applying Adaptive Design

When should you use Adaptive Design (AD)? It depends on the problem.

TYPES OF PROBLEMS	PROBLEM DEFINITION	PROBLEM SOLUTION	EXAMPLES	USE AD?
I. Technical	Clear	Clear	Picking instruments for or doing an appendectomy. Initiating therapy for diabetes.	No
II. Complex Technical	Clear	Difficult to define, complex, interdependent	Building a new operating room. Severe trauma. Diabetic ketoacidosis.	Optional
III. Adaptive	Unclear, many potential causes, chaotic, variable inputs and/or outputs	Ill-defined, cause and effect, unpredictable, complex, variable, chaotic	Improving OR productivity. Changing habits, behaviors and values of people. Raising a child.	Yes

In Adaptive Design, senior leadership gets off the fire-fighting/meeting treadmill and starts to develop and exert its real authority.

Leadership is a journey. The great leadership challenge of healthcare is that it is naturally complex, dynamic and unpredictable. What do we really know about tomorrow? When facing the facts, we can only admit, "We know we don't know!" That's a problem in a planned and implemented world, because the safe path keeps changing in unknown and unknowable ways.

However, with Adaptive Design the journey is not a chaotic, unpredictable wilderness. Instead, the path has guideposts, milestones and, most importantly, a built-in way to respond:

- The **direction** is toward Ideal Patient Care.
- We are **protected** from unexpected changes by tested, validated, improvable ways to quickly respond. And it is always safe to challenge the status quo.
- We have a safe method to respond because senior **management creates order**, clarity and consistency with a set of rules, skills and tools that generate results.
- Results come from **decision-making** that follows the rules and makes it safe to move toward Ideal Patient Care.

And now the loop is back to Ideal. We just repeat what we now know how to do.

Management learns, leads, teaches and challenges cycles of increasing returns. The people in the organization learn, respond and deliver for their patients and co-workers. Patient care moves toward Ideal.

It is a different way to work.

GOLD AND WISDOM

"[T]he method of Hippocrates is the only method that has ever succeeded widely and generally [in accomplishing change and improvement in healthcare]. The first element of that method is hard, persistent, intelligent, responsible, unremitting labor in the sick room, not in the library."

– LAWRENCE JOSEPH HENDERSON

As stated in the Prologue, this book is about leading in challenging times.

In this turbulent decade, leaders in healthcare have understandably looked outside of the medical profession for answers:

Perhaps hopes lie in a national, single-payer health system for the U.S.

Maybe computers, advanced information technologies, state-of-the-art diagnostic systems and the latest management tools and methods will rescue us.

Perhaps the promulgation of more guidelines, best practices and evidenced-based medicine will provide the solution.

Or, perhaps these are all just wild hopes and impossible dreams.

On the frontlines, healthcare workers are pessimistic and they are increasingly voting with their feet by leaving the profession.

Me – I'm optimistic. If there is a single message in this book, it is that the solutions to the healthcare challenges of today and tomorrow lie deep within each organization – like gold, waiting to be mined.

Perhaps our outdated ways of "prospecting" are what make the treasure so hard to identify and discover. Just like the treasure of the Sierra Madre.

You may remember the 1940s classic film, *The Treasure of the Sierra Madre*, starring Humphrey Bogart. The movie has many wonderful scenes about the human propensity to misapprehend value or overlook it entirely, even when it lays in plain sight.

The movie itself is a nugget worth watching. Three down-and-outers take-up prospecting and strike-out into the uncharted mountains of Mexico to find their fortune in gold. After weeks of trudging through inhospitable terrain, Fred C. Dobbs (Bogart) and his greenhorn sidekick, Curtin, discover what they think is the "mother lode" in boulders strewn about in the arid foothills.

But reality dumps cold water on their fired-up hopes when the third partner, Howard, a wise old-timer (played by Walter Huston, who won the Academy Award that year for best supporting actor), sadly informs them that the glittering metal in the rocks is only "pyrite... fool's gold."

Later, as the trio ascends even higher into the mountains, Dobbs and Curtin sit exhausted in the dirt, discouraged and ready to call it quits. Suddenly Howard starts a mad little jig, kicking up the dust and delivering a soliloquy that's as close to Shakespearian as Hollywood ever gets.

The other two, he mocks, are no more than "two shoe clerks readin' a magazine about prospecting." They are blind to the riches under their own sorry feet. Howard, the *wisest* prospector, has been seeing the signs for days – there's real gold in these mountains.

You just have to know how to find it!

In every healthcare system I have visited, the greatest treasure is the people. *People are the gold!* Only with them and through them can institutions learn how to develop higher quality, more responsive, safer patient care – at lower cost.

Looking at healthcare's future through the lens of Adaptive Design, the financial opportunities are not only more understandable, they are completely predictable.

Success clearly depends on adapting for the future. Metaphorically "mining the gold" involves switching the focus from external funding to internal development. For example, **I can guarantee** that in the next decade the most successful healthcare organizations will have a financial strategy starkly opposed to their competition in five ways, by:

1. Excelling at Return on Assets instead of Return on Investment,
2. Regenerating capital rather than accessing and expending capital,
3. Problem solving with ingenuity rather than technology,
4. Creating new best practices instead of copying someone else's, and
5. Developing people — not things — as the organization's number 1 resource.

How to create these differences is simple, but not easy. Although much knowledge is at work in healthcare, the system is still out of balance. Knowledge must be balanced by wisdom, *internal* wisdom. There is no other option. Restore the balance by capturing the knowledge, creativity, problem solving ability and wisdom of everyone in the organization — *Everyone*! What fool would mine one nugget — and leave the rest lying?

Adaptive Design restores the balance by developing people. People are our number 1 resource, the "gold" that is all around us. (Leaders are discovering that — and doing the jig!)

Adaptive Design develops people through discipline, structure and problem solving when systems fail to meet patient needs Ideally.

Adaptive Design captures and develops the knowledge, creativity and problem solving ability of every person in the organization toward a common purpose.

Adaptive Design uses that common purpose to focus on just one thing — Ideal Patient Care.

Adaptive Design gives management new clarity, consistency and authenticity by tying their work to developing and challenging problem solving at the point-of-care.

Adaptive Design drives out the crippling effects of ambiguity, assumptions, workarounds and tradeoffs.

Adaptive Design changes expectations. Remember the comment of Jane RN at St. TAH's: "We became intolerant of mediocrity."

Adaptive Design captures the knowledge *and* the wisdom that resides in people to restore balance in healthcare.

Adaptive Design gets patients exactly what they need at continually lower cost.

Wisdom in action — that's Adaptive Design. There is no other way for healthcare to successfully face the challenges of today and those in the years ahead.

Now is the time and the time is now! It's the way to fix healthcare!

A SELECTED, ANNOTATED
BIBLIOGRAPHY

Chapter 1: The Climb

Tucker, A. L., & Edmondson, A. C. (2003). Why Hospitals Don't Learn from Failures: Organizational and Psychological Dynamics that Inhibit System Change. *California Management Review, 45*(2), 55 – 72.

This article is one of the two key articles used to teach problem solving in the course of work. Most readers will relate to the dilemma that the authors introduce:

- Problems (not errors) make the difference at the point-of-care,
- First-order problem solving is a proudly worn "badge of honor" in healthcare, but it also contributes significantly to the "dynamics that inhibit system change."

Chapter 2: Why Toyota?

Ohno, T. (1988). *Toyota Production System: Beyond Large-Scale Production.* New York, NY: Productivity Press.

Ohno's is the classic description of the Toyota Production System, written by an insider who was part of the development of the Toyota Way. He makes his point right in the title and repeats in the first three pages of the book: TPS is not about maximizing profit through economies of scale, but rather having the flexibility to profitably make small numbers of many different products. Developing that flexibility led to Toyota's transition from industrial management to knowledge management.

Takeuchi, H., Osono, E., & Shimizu, N. (2008). *Extreme Toyota: Radical Contradictions That Drive Success at the World's Best Manufacturer.* Hoboken, NJ: John Wiley & Sons.

This recent book does a much better job of outlining and analyzing Toyota's unique management methods than most books that approach Toyota through a process-improvement point of view.

Von Hayek, F.A. (1945). The use of Knowledge in Society. Institute for Humane Studies, Inc., Menlo Park, CA 94025. Reprint No. 5.

Few scholars in the 20th Century have equaled the breadth of Friedrich A. von Hayek's interests in the humane sciences. This is a slightly revised and abbreviated version of an article that first appeared in *The American Economic Review*. Vol. 35, No. 4, September 1945. Although the paper focuses on economic systems as a whole (Hayek predicts the crash of planned economies 40 years before it happened), it's the first, and maybe one of the best, "knowledge management" papers I have seen.

Chapter 4: A Demand for Change

Collins, J. (2001). *Good to Great: Why Some Companies Make the Leap... and Others Don't.* New York, NY: HarperCollins Publishers, Inc.

Obviously a classic for many reasons, the attributes of *Good to Great* that Collins documents fit Adaptive Design very well. Collins identifies *what to do*; Adaptive Design provides the *how*.

Chapter 5: Disruptive Innovation: To Stop the Machine

All of Clayton Christensen's writings can be applied to Adaptive Design in one way or another. Many have a pessimistic view of hospitals and current healthcare methods, while I am optimistic that Adaptive Design will give a few established organizations the power to make a difference and lead the way.

Christensen, C. M. (1997). *The Innovator's Dilemma: The Revolutionary Book That Will Change the Way You Do Business*. Boston, MA: Harvard Business School Press.

Clayton Christensen's first book is the classic description of disruptive innovation – the kind of innovation that leading companies find almost impossible to do.

Christensen, C. M., Bohmer, R., & Kenagy, J. (2000, Sept – Oct.). Will Disruptive Innovations Cure Health Care? *Harvard Business Review*, 102 – 111.

This article is the first description of disruptive innovation in healthcare.

Christensen, C. M., Baumann, H., Ruggles, R., & Sadtler, T. (2006, Dec.). Disruptive Innovation for Social Change. *Harvard Business Review*. 94 – 101.

A recent review of disruptive innovation with reference to healthcare that reiterates the fact that established organizations find it "almost impossible" to disrupt themselves.

Christensen, C. M., & Overdorf, M. (2000, Mar – Apr). Meeting the Challenge of Disruptive Change. *Harvard Business Review*. 67 – 76.

It may be "almost impossible," but this article is particularly good at outlining how established organizations can expand the possible and create and execute a disruptive strategy. It influenced the development of many of the skills and tools of Adaptive Design.

Christensen, C. M., Grossman, J., & Hwang, J. (2009). *The Innovator's Prescription: A Disruptive Solution for Health Care*. New York, NY: McGraw-Hill.

Christensen's new book on the disruption of healthcare is essential reading to *anyone* interested in innovation and management in healthcare.

Chandler, A. D. (1977). *The Visible Hand: The Managerial Revolution in American Business*. Cambridge, MA: Belknap Press of Harvard University Press.

This business history classic details the rise of the professional managerial hierarchy in the late 19th and early 20th Century capitalism. It was invaluable in helping me understand our current management methods – what I have come to call the Traditional Business Enterprise.

Chapter 6: Adaptive Design in Practice: The Rules-In-Use

Spear, S. J., & Bowen, H. K. (1999). Decoding the DNA of the Toyota Production System. *Harvard Business Review*. 96 – 106.

> The second key article — one of the two cornerstones on which Adaptive Design is built and an exposition of a brilliant piece of investigative research. A Tokyo University business school professor told me that, of all the hundreds of books and articles written about Toyota, this is one of only two that Toyota has translated into Japanese.

Spear, S. J., & Kenagy, J. (2005). Deaconess-Glover Hospital. *Harvard Business School Case Study*. 9-601-022.

> This is a Harvard Business School Teaching Case detailing the first use of TPS and the first application of Rules-In Use in healthcare. These healthcare cases have been taught at Harvard and other academic institutions, and in many industries including at Toyota, itself.

Chapter 7: Rule 4: Creating IDEAL Healthcare

Fishman, C. (2006, Dec.). No Satisfaction at Toyota. *Fast Company*. 82.

> In my experience, most of the articles written about Toyota in the popular and business press just simply "don't get it." The framework that Toyota works with is just too different from conventional business practices. Fishman gets it. This is the best article I have read on Toyota for the general reader. Highly recommended.

Christensen, C. M., & Sundahl, D. (1991). The Process of Building Theory. *Harvard Business School Working Paper*. 02-016.

> This Harvard Business School Working Paper will help those who want to know more about applying the Scientific Method and developing new theory for how and why things work (or don't work). It may not be easy to obtain, but I will be happy to send a copy to anyone who requests it. Contact me at john@johnkenagy.com.

Jimmerson, C. (2007). *A3 Problem Solving for Healthcare: A Practical Method for Eliminating Waste*. New York, NY: Productivity Press.

This is an excellent and practical guide to using A3s and clearly one of the best Lean healthcare books. Highly recommended.

Chapter 8: Harnessing the Power of Continuous Innovation

McCraw, T. K. (2007). *Prophet of Innovation: Joseph Schumpeter and Creative Destruction*. Cambridge, MA: Harvard Business School Publishing.

Schumpeter's "Creative Destruction" is an obvious predecessor to Christensen's much more thorough study of disruptive innovation. McCraw's biography is a well-told story of a fascinating man, *bon vivant* and economic scholar who discovered the fact that successful companies are, at times, their own worst enemies.

Seligman, M. (1998). *Learned Optimism: How to Change Your Mind and Your Life*. New York, NY: Simon and Schuster.

Seligman's work has been a revelation to those of us doing Adaptive Design. "Optimism, pessimism and learned helplessness," all of Seligman's insights apply to 21st Century healthcare.

Senge, P. M. (2006). *The Fifth Discipline: The Art & Practice of the Learning Organization*. New York, NY: Random House.

This is the classic "learning organization" reference. A recent article on the subject with great application to healthcare is:

Garvin, D. A., Edmondson, A. C., & Gino, F. (2008, March). Is Yours a Learning Organization? *Harvard Business Review*, R0803H.

Chapter 9: "Getting It Done:" Real-Time Lessons from Adaptive Organizations

Braaten, J. S., & Bellhouse, D. E. (2007). Improving Patient Care by Making Small Sustainable Changes: A Cardiac Telemetry Unit's Experience. *Nursing Economic$*, (25)3, 162 – 166.

This article is the first case study description of Adaptive Design and problem solving in the course of work in the medical literature. This is a pioneering, perhaps classic, article.

Chapter 10: A New Way of Seeing: A New Way of Leading

Spear, S. J. (2004, May). Learning to Lead at Toyota. *Harvard Business Review*. 78 – 86.

> Another Spear classic that not only details the baptism of an "American hot-shot" manager in the deep waters of the Toyota Production System, but also makes it clear what the differences are between traditional, industrial-styled management and Toyota's knowledge management system. I use this article as a foundation in developing the Management Learning Line.

Heifetz, R. A. (1994). *Leadership Without Easy Answers*. Cambridge, MA: The Belknap Press of Harvard University Press.

> In the Prologue, I mentioned "common threads" of thinking weaving through many different authors' works. Well, truth be told, "adaptive" came from Ron Heifetz's concept of technical and adaptive problem solving in leadership. His work has had significant influence on these concepts. I have turned back to this book many times in my research, teaching and mentoring work with senior management.

More common threads — not referred to in the book but part of the fabric...

Spear, S. J. (2008). *Chasing the Rabbit: How Market Leaders Outdistance the Competition and How Great Companies Can Catch Up and Win*. New York, NY: McGraw-Hill.

> Just as this book is being finished, Spear has published this summary of his experience. I believe Spear to be the world's expert on managing collaborative work in a complex, dynamic, unpredictable environment and highly recommended this book to you.

Balik, Barbara; Nyberg, Amy; Andersohn, Wendi; Knudtson, Barbara; Gardner, Diane; Lambert, Mary; Heichert, Susan; Werni, Susan, Tina. *Workflows & the Electronic Health Record: Applying Toyota Principles to Improve Implementation*, (in preparation for publication).

Each of these authors is a true Adaptive Design pioneer and expert. In my view, their work helps develop the framework for an extremely valuable application of these concepts in healthcare information systems.

Kuhn, T. (1996). *The Structure of Scientific Revolutions. (3rd Edition).* Chicago, IL: The University of Chicago Press.

A classic in science history, Kuhn beautifully develops how the leaders of the "current science" are almost always the last to accept a new paradigm, the "new science." It's disruptive innovation all over again in different clothes.

Baldwin, C. Y., & Clark, K. B. (2000). *Design Rules: The Power of Modularity.* Cambridge, MA: MIT Press.

"Modularity" is a powerful concept I did not mention in this book, but fundamental to many of Adaptive Design's ideas, methods and success. Put in Baldwin and Clark's framework, Toyota is a "nested modular system" and the Rules-In-Use are "design rules." This book is essential reading for those who want to go deeper into adaptive work methods.

Argyris, C. S. (1991, May – June). Teaching Smart People How to Learn. *Harvard Business Review.* 99 – 109.

Chris Argyris is another Harvard icon whose work has influenced many people at HBS, including Bowen and Spear. In this article, he first makes the point that it can be difficult to get smart people to learn (they "already know"), and then develops a logical approach to "teaching smart people how to learn." This is essential reading for those who must try to teach doctors and senior managers to learn.

Von Hippel, E. (2005). *Democratizing Innovation.* Cambridge, MA: MIT Press.

MIT Professor Von Hippel takes another approach to the power of frontline learning and describes how the base of the organization, not the top, commonly is the source of groundbreaking innovation. I just wish I had thought of the name "democratizing innovation" first — evocative and right on the money.

Tushman, M. L., & O'Reilly, C. A. (1996). The Ambidextrous Organization: Managing Evolutionary and Revolutionary Change. *California Management Review*, 38(4), 8 – 30.

> We commonly use this excellent article with senior management on the Management Learning Line. The authors eloquently make the case for separation of innovative efforts within a larger organization and emphasize how to do that safely.

Kotter, J. (1955, March – April). Leading Change: Why Transformation Efforts Fail. *Harvard Business Review*. 59 – 67.

> A business classic that looks at change from the viewpoint of transforming an entire organization. This is another popular article on the Management Learning Line.

Kaplan, R. (1998). Innovation Action Research: Creating New Management Theory and Practice. *Journal of Management Accounting Research*. 10, 89 – 117.

> Harvard Business School Professor Robert Kaplan, the creator of the Balanced Scorecard, kindly introduced me to this paper. Action-Innovation Research is the model I have followed in creating Adaptive Design.

Johnson, S. (2001). *Emergence: The Connected Lives of Ants, Brains, Cities, and Software*. New York, NY: Scribner.

> Johnson could have added hospitals and health systems to his "connected lives." Healthcare systems are, in Johnson's parlance, complex, adaptive systems. And they can follow rules. Emergence of clarity out of chaos is the story of rule-based, self-organizing systems and Adaptive Design in healthcare. This book is both a readable and instructive journey through emergence theory, feedback, self-organization and adaptive learning.

AN ADAPTIVE GLOSSARY

A3 — An 11X17 piece of paper and a specified method to design, test and validate all changes in Adaptive Design as experiments. A3s are composed of six elements:

1. Background
2. Current Condition
3. Root Cause
4. Target Condition
5. Countermeasures
6. Test

Activities — The work of a single person or the specified work of a small group of people to create a specific outcome or objective. Rule 1 of the Rules-In-Use states that Activities are specified as to content, sequence, timing and outcome.

Adaptive Design — A set of methods, skills and tools designed to get healthcare back to the ideals of patient care by cultivating adaptability in the everyday work of the organization and it's people. Adaptive Design brings science to the workplace to continually improve an organization's ability to deliver exactly what a patient needs at continually lower cost. It does so by creating self-diagnostic and self-improving systems embedded into everyday work and developing people as the organization's number one resource. It's a way for everyone to see, do and improve, everywhere, everyday. It's the way to fix healthcare.

Background — The initial element in an A3 that establishes the business case and identifies the problem. Often written "Ideally... but the problem is..."

Best Practice — Tied to evidence-based medicine, best practice can describe specific expectations for good patient care. For example, diabetic patients should measure blood sugar and many elderly patients should have flu shots. That we can all understand. From the Adaptive Design point-of-view, the problem is when these "best practices" become rigid mandates and dogma. Yes, *most* elderly patients, but not all, should have flu vaccine and *how* that will happen is highly dependent on the context of the Current Condition, both very adaptive problems.

Connections — Describes how two people connect to create value. Rule 2 of the Rules-In-Use states that all Connections are simple, direct and have an unambiguous yes/no way to send requests and receive responses.

Countermeasures — The fifth element of an A3 that describes the steps we will take to move from the problematic Current Condition to the solution in the Target Condition.

Current Condition — The second element of an A3 that graphically and pictorially represents the way we currently work and the problem that work caused.

Disruptive Innovation — An innovation characteristically based on simple technology meeting the unmet needs of a group of customers that are not on the "radar screen" of leading, established organizations. The innovation then improves to allow many appropriately skilled, more accessible, lower cost people to do the work of centralized, expensive specialists. Most established leading organizations find it almost impossible to disrupt their current business models. Adaptive Design seeks to expand the possible for healthcare.

Error — The execution of a task that was either unnecessary or incorrectly carried out.

First-Order Problem Solving — Taking the measures necessary to compensate for a problem without undertaking the steps to assure that the failure or problem will not occur again.

Help Chain — A vertical slice of the organization that connects the front-line worker to the most senior manager in the organization. Problems rise in the Help Chain only as high as they need to go to achieve a testable, verifiable solution.

Ideal Patient Care — The "North Star" that sets direction in Adaptive Design:
- Exactly what patients need, when and where they need it;
- Customized individually;
- Immediate response to problems or changes;
- Safe — physically, emotionally and professionally — for patients, staff, management and clinicians;
- Without waste of any resource.

"I have a problem" — The key signal that current work does not meet patient, staff, clinician or management needs Ideally. Always signaled to a specified person as close in time and place to the problem as possible.

Knowledge Worker — The classic definition is "one who works primarily with information or one who develops knowledge in the workplace." It is usually ascribed to people who work in information technology or more traditionally creative places than assembly lines. Manufacturing workers are essentially never classified as "knowledge workers" — except by Toyota. Toyota's marvelous insight that valuable information is embedded into the work of almost everyone on an assembly line is an entirely new perspective- a new *gestalt* — on the nature of work. If there is value in considering people on an assembly line as knowledge workers, consider the power of the concept in healthcare.

Learner/Leader/Teacher — The title of the first Adaptive Design learners in the organization. This term ultimately describes the work of all managers and, ideally, many of the workers in the organization.

Learning Line — A specified group of people, technologies, equipment and/or supplies who come together to create a good or service that can be isolated to create an environment for adaptive problem solving. The Learning Line environment is designed to foster trust, optimism, high performance and innovation. Ideally, it is a relatively simple pathway (see Rules-In-Use) creating meaningful goods or services for the organization. "Small, simple and separate" are the key words. Learning Lines create the opportunity to learn-by-doing Adaptive Design.

Management Learning Line — The frontline has a great advantage over management in Adaptive Design because they have a safe place to learn-the Learning Line. Just as this book is being written, the first Management Learning Lines are being developed. This is the new frontier for adaptive work in healthcare.

Pathways — How many people, supplies, technologies and other things come together to create complex goods and services. Rule 3 states: All pathways are simple, direct and include all the elements necessary (and no element unnecessary) to create a good or service.

Power Chains — Simple pathways from the CEO to the frontline not only create Help Chains, they create Power Chains for senior management to increasingly match accountability and control on the frontline to move patient care toward Ideal.

Problem — A disruption in the worker's ability to execute a prescribed task because either what was needed was unavailable or something got in the way.

Problem Solving — Rule 4 in the Rules-In-Use states that problems are solved under the guidance of a teacher using the Scientific Method as close in time and place to the problem as possible.

Root Cause — The third element of an A3 that seeks to identify the underlying cause of the problem illustrated in the Current Condition. The Root Cause is commonly identified by asking "Why," five times. The Root Cause is often characterized by one of the first three Rules-In-Use.

Rules-In-Use — The four unwritten, unspoken, but generally followed rules (discovered by Steven Spear and H. Kent Bowen) that govern the work of the frontline and management at Toyota. The Rules govern Activities, Connections, Pathways and Problem Solving. These rules are a fundamental part of Toyota's DNA that creates their capability to be "designed to adapt" and are also fundamental to Adaptive Design.

Second-Order Problem Solving — Taking the measures necessary to compensate for a problem and also systematically addressing the Root Cause of the problem to eliminate its recurrence, resulting in work-process improvement and institutional learning.

Specified Problem-Solver — The person (Learner/Leader/Teacher) specified for a defined group of people that facilitates problem solving as close in time and place to the problem as possible.

Target Condition — The fourth element of an A3 that pictorially and graphically shows a new way to work in which the problem would not occur.

Test — The sixth element of an A3 that determines (Yes/No) if the Target Condition was achieved. If the Test is "Yes," and the Target Condition is stable, the A3 is complete. If it is "No," or the Target Condition is not stable, that is a problem to solve.

ACKNOWLEDGEMENTS

Adaptive Design is learning-by-doing, and "doing" is rarely a solitary activity in modern healthcare. The concepts outlined in this book are the sum of more than 40 years of my own doing and learning at the point-of-care. As such, literally hundreds of people contributed to these pages — teachers, mentors, colleagues, friends, family and patients. To those my poor memory has undoubtedly missed, I offer my sincere apologies.

All physicians are influenced by their education. I was uncommonly fortunate to attend the University of Nebraska for both undergraduate studies and medical school. I have since been in many academic institutions and not yet discovered one that could equal the patient-focused, clinical education I was so fortunate to receive from the University of Nebraska, College of Medicine, in Omaha.

I am convinced that my surgical residency training and subsequent clinical faculty work in Seattle at the University of Washington (UW) were formative not only to my clinical skills but also to my earliest adaptive learning. Doctors Eugene Strandness, Malcolm Perry, Tom Marchioro, Jim Carrico, Dave Heimbach, Tom Shires, Ron Maier, Michael Copass and Hugh Foy were particularly influential in my development. They set the tone, and Gene Strandness was the first true disruptive innovator I ever met, long before the term was coined. I am proud to remain a Clinical Associate Professor of Surgery at UW and greatly appreciate the support and guidance Surgery Chairman Carlos Pelligrini, MD, has generously offered over the years.

Longview, Washington, was my next stop — for 20 years. Doctors Roger Grummel and Mel Ofstun invited me to join their practice, and a fledging surgeon could not have been more fortunate. The concept of Ideal Patient Care grew from the example set for me by Roger, Mel, and my other partners and associates including Diane Smith and all our wonderful staff at Longview Surgical Group. George Fortner, MD, deserves special mention as the person who seamlessly took over a two-man vascular surgery practice when one half of the team fell out of a tree and broke his neck.

Breaking my neck gave me an unintended but very unique view of healthcare. Fortunately, I worked with a healthcare system, PeaceHealth, in which others could share that view. Many leaders within PeaceHealth accepted and vigorously encouraged my interests. It was the nature of the organization and their founders, the Sisters of St. Joseph of Peace, to take a stand and do something different. What they did different for me was to accept, engage and support a not very hospital business-savvy surgeon in learning the ways of healthcare management in real-time. Many, many people helped and encouraged me to make this transition. Again, I cannot list all the names but Sister Eleanor Gilmore, Sister Anne Hayes and Sister Monique Herron stand out among many others. PeaceHealth carries out the Mission of their sponsors; they mean what they say.

One more Longview person needs to be mentioned – Jim Meskew. Jim worked to develop vascular radiology at St. Johns Hospital; helped create one of healthcare's first private practice, non-invasive vascular laboratories; took the lead management position at Longview Surgery and eventually become Chief Operating Officer for St. Johns Medical Center. Remarkable accomplishments all, but most important to me, he continues to be a guide and a friend. That's a wonderful combination.

Then to Harvard, where Dr. Miles Shore's course, "Understanding the New World of Health Care" at the Kennedy School of Government (KSG), ignited my enthusiasm to look outside of healthcare. Miles was key to my making the decision to take "just one year off" and enter KSG's Mid-Career Master of Public Administration program. Miles also influenced my view of leadership. I will always remember his insight that "all change is a loss," and his admonition that "the change agent must also appreciate and support the grieving of those undergoing change."

The Kennedy School Mid-Career MPA program was an amazing experience for a 50-year-old surgeon wondering why it was so tough to manage healthcare. My classmates, a skilled, experienced, diverse group from the U.S. and 40 other countries, taught me that we learn from each other, as well as the professors. I cannot name all the people who made a difference, but one professor stands out: Ron Heifetz, MD. His concept of technical and adaptive leadership is part of the bedrock of Adaptive Design. Every day I use what I learned from him.

Next to Harvard Business School where Professor Clayton Christensen stretched my brain into a new place with his concept of disruptive innovation. Fortunately, he was bold enough to invite onboard a vascular surgeon as a Visiting Scholar at Harvard Business School to help develop on the concept of disruptive innovation in healthcare. And from that came this work. Clay has remained a continual source of new ideas, support and a true friend. With disruptive innovation, he created the framework and common language that grew into the strategic aspects of Adaptive Design.

In addition, Clay introduced me to Harvard Business School Professors Steve Spear and Kent Bowen. Kent and Steve were willing to take on a physician who thought that Toyota's Rules-In-Use might fit the complex, dynamic world of healthcare. Through the first two years of my learning, they continually supported and challenged me. Along with Clay, they helped me connect the dots from theory to practical improvement in healthcare. And, in addition, they introduced me directly to key Toyota personnel.

I am particularly indebted to Carolyn Schindley-Parker and Hajime Ohba of the Toyota Supplier Support Center who graciously gave me their time and provided learning opportunities.

Harvard Business School Professors Regina Herzlinger (healthcare economics), Jim Heskett (service quality) and Bob Kaplan (innovation-action research) were all very generous with their ideas, time and support in the development of these concepts. Finally, the unique work and insights of Professor Chris Argyris are common threads that run throughout the fabric of Adaptive Design.

That covers the beginnings of Adaptive Design. The conclusion will never be written, because it will never stop being improved by the people who do the work. From the beginning, I have been blessed to associate with great people in doing Adaptive Design. Since "learning-by-doing" is key, the people who have practiced Adaptive Design have been central to the development of these ideas.

First and foremost are all those who worked for and partnered with me in advising and consulting in healthcare, beginning with Kenagy & Associates, LLC, and Rule 4 Consulting: David Sundahl, PhD, Jon Roberts, Dorothy (Dolly) Bellhouse, Jimmy Udall, Jameson Rehm, Deborah Burkholder, Monique Doyle and Pam Linder, RN.

And Cambridge Management Group: Bob Harrington, Jim Dorsey, Andy Nighswander and Ken Cohn, MD.

But consultants and advisors need to work with people who actually do the work. When I say Adaptive Design is a product of the people who do the work, I mean it. These are a few of the key people in the development of Adaptive Design and the institutions that supported their and our work:

Beth Israel Deaconess Medical Center, Boston, MA and Deaconess Glover Hospital (now Beth Israel Deaconess — Needham), Needham, MA: John Dalton, Julie Bonnefant and James Reinertsen, MD.

Pittsburgh Regional Healthcare Initiative and University of Pittsburgh Medical Center, Pittsburgh, PA: Randy Smith, Bob Weber, Paul O'Neil, Lisa Beckwith, Gail Wolf, Debra Thompson, Karen Feinstein and Ken Segel.

St. Johns Hospital, Jackson, WY: Jonathan Schechter, Ron Ommen and Jayne Ottman, RN.

Microsoft, Redmond, WA: David Lubinski, Bill Crounse, MD, and Christine Williams.

Johns Hopkins University, Baltimore, MD: Richard (Chip) Davis, PhD.

Institute for Healthcare Improvement, Boston, MA: Don Berwick, MD.

Porter Adventist Hospital, Centura Health, Denver, CO: Joe Swedish, Amy Nyberg, John Burns, Lyn Mathias, RN, Jim Boyle, Claudia Stafford, Sheri Clark, RN; Jane Braaten, RN, Carol Hickman, Paul Reeder and Sharon Pappas, PhD.

Cambridge Health Alliance, Cambridge, MA: Edward Dunn, MD, Jeffery Steinberg, MD, Dennis Keefe, Kevin Kelley, Linda Nelson, Suzie Rhodes, Lisa O'Connor, Warren Rhodes, Jimmy Mello, Paul Vibol, Sam Doppelt, MD, and Iris Box.

Allina Health and Hospital System's many executives, managers and nurses supported Adaptive Design's development, including: Barbara Balik, Kathy Wilde, Venetia Kuderle, Amy Nyberg, Margo Watkins, RN, Wendi Andersohn, RN, Wendy Larkin, RN, Bonnie Mehrer, RN, Diane Gardner, RN, Connie Fiebiger, RN, Kathy Shields Kupfer, Colin Baird, Shelly Sampson, RN, Mary Lambert, Barb Knutdson, Megha Mungekar and David Dooher.

National Hospice Work Group: True Ryndes, David Rehm and Don Schumacher

Hospice of the Western Reserve, Cleveland, OH: David Simpson, Shareefah Sabur, Melissa Sommer, Florence and Andy Luptak.

Continuum Hospice, New York City: Katherine Brown and Carolyn Cassin.

VNSNY Hospice, New York City, NY: Pat Vigilante, RN.

Ascension Health, St. Louis, MO: Hyung Kim, MD, Anthony Tersigni, John Doyle, Bob Henkle, Eric Engler, Peggy Kurusz, Sister Maureen McGuire and Matt Hermann.

St. Vincent's Health, Indianapolis, IN: Vince Caponi, LouAnne Crawley Stout, Kathy Young, and John Rahman, MD.

St Vincent Randolph: Frank Albarino, Carla Fouse, RN, Nicole Pegg, RN.

St. Joseph Hospital, Kokomo, IN: Darcy Burthay, RN, Mary Ellen Griffin, Jennifer Lefler, RN, Kim Shepherd, RN, Laura Caulfield, Tony Kinney and Joe Klein.

Seton Hospital, Indianapolis, IN: Peter Alexander, Troy Reiff, Melanie Holt, Dave Girten, Angie Hagan, Kristina Patterson and Joe Morrow.

PHNS, Dallas, TX: Richard Kneipper.

Palomar Pomerado Health, San Diego, CA: Michael Covert, Carrie Frederick, Natalie Bennett, Steve Vannoy, Gerald Bracht, Bruce Grendell, RN, Lori Shoemaker, RN, PhD, David Tam, Duane Buringrud, MD, Sheila Brown, Kimberley Dotson, RN, MBA and Marcia Jackson.

Mayo Health System: Particular thanks to Mark Lindsay, MD, Brian Bunkers, MD, and Kathy Huttar, RN, for initiating adaptive work in Mayo; and to all the MHS Learner/Leader/Teachers and Management Learning Line: Jim Haemmerle, MD, Tamra Albers, Lesa Anderson, David Beckmann, MD, David Berg, Lee Boettcher, Pat Buretta, Molly Cain, Mark Ciota, MD, Debra Degrood, Jeannie Green, John Grzybowski, Gayle Hansen, David Hellstern, Mary Huepfel, Mary Kerg, Virginia (Ginny) Larson, RN, Tonia Lauer, Steven Lindberg, Darren Lokkesmoe, MD, Cynthia Muth, Karl Palmer, RN, Terri Peterson, MD, Reinhold Plate, MD, Stephen Pribyl, Carol Rypka, Mary Simms Sheehan, Henry (Hank) Simpson, MD, Bridget Strand, Philip Vuocolo, MD, Stephen Waldhoff, Jody Wright, RN, Jody Hauser, RN and Shari Kropp.

The list could go on and on. Doubtless, I have not included everyone, but I do know we could not have done it without these and many others.

Books require writing, and I am indebted to S. Harvey Price for asking me to write for his healthcare CEO newsletter, *For Your Advantage*. Jerry Pogue, the publisher of Second River Healthcare Press, has encouraged this work from the beginning. Chris Jackson, also of Second River Healthcare Press, was instrumental in bringing this book to fruition.

Michael Melford has offered sage legal advice and the support as a good friend throughout this endeavor. Finally, the work of an entrepreneur is strange business for a doc; Richard (Dick) Sass has provided me the real-life model and freely given me his advice, counsel and friendship for many years.

But writing is where the rubber meets the road, and without the talent, editing and rewriting support provided by Michelle Nash and John Read, this book would never have reached its final form.

Finally and most importantly, thanks to family. They have followed and supported me wherever this endeavor has taken us over the last 12 years. Lisa Day Sandstrom, in particular, has given me support and freely offered her talents as an artist and film editor to Adaptive Design. But, it's the immediate family that deserves the final accolades. I am sure they will be the first to say, "The transformation of healthcare is not easy!" Jonell, Jen Aroha, Susanne, Emma and John-thanks for all your help, support, forbearance, fortitude and love. It would never have happened without you.